Pediatric Drug Formulations

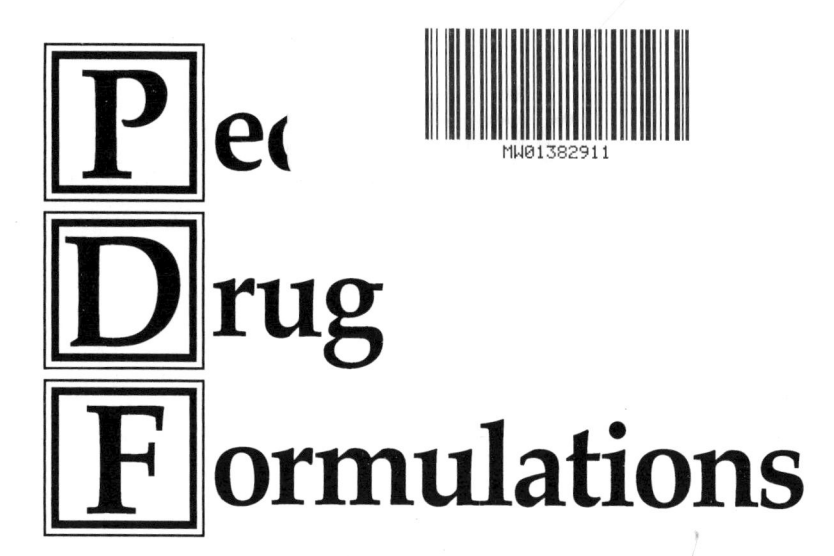

Sixth Edition

Milap C. Nahata, Pharm.D.
Professor of Pharmacy and Pediatrics
Colleges of Pharmacy and Medicine
The Ohio State University
Children's Hospital
Columbus, Ohio

Vinita B. Pai, Pharm.D.
Assistant Professor
College of Pharmacy
The Ohio State University

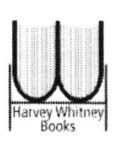

HARVEY WHITNEY BOOKS COMPANY
CINCINNATI, OHIO USA

Copyright © 2011
Harvey Whitney Books Company
4906 Cooper Rd., P.O. Box 42696
Cincinnati, OH 45242 USA
www.hwbooks.com

All rights reserved. Reproduction or translation of any part of this work beyond that permitted by Sections 107 or 108 of the 1976 United States Copyright Act without permission of the copyright owner is unlawful. No part of this publication may be utilized by any information storage and retrieval system, or transmitted, in any form or by any means, electronic, mechanical, photocopying, recording, or otherwise, without prior written permission from the publisher.

First Edition © 1990
Second Edition © 1992
Third Edition © 1997
Fourth Edition © 2000
Fifth Edition © 2003
Fifth Edition, Revised and Reprinted © 2004
Sixth Edition © 2011

The information contained in this publication is intended to supplement the knowledge of healthcare professionals regarding pediatric drug formulations. The publisher disclaims any warranty as to the quality, accuracy, or suitability of this information, and assumes no responsibility for any injury and/or damage to persons from the use of any methods, instructions, or ideas contained in the material herein.

The information provided is not intended to be interpreted as a substitute for the official compendia, such as the *United States Pharmacopeia*.

Printed in the United States of America

International Standard Book Number: 0-929375-32-8

Table of Contents

Preface to the Sixth Edition	xi
Preface to the Fifth Edition	xiii
Preface to the Fourth Edition	xiv
Preface to the Third Edition	xv
Preface to the Second Edition	xvi
Preface to the First Edition	xviii
Introduction to the Formulations	1

Formulations

Acetazolamide (oral suspension, solution)
Acetylcysteine (oral solution, ophthalmic solution)
Adderall (oral suspension)
Allopurinol (oral suspension)
Alprazolam (oral suspension)
Amiloride (oral suspension)
Aminophylline (injection)
5-Aminosalicylic Acid enema (suspension)
Amiodarone (oral suspension)
Amitriptyline (oral suspension, oral liquid)
Amlodipine (oral suspension)
Amphotericin B (nasal solution, oral suspension)
Aprepitant (oral suspension)
Atenolol (oral suspension)
Atropine Sulfate (injection, oral solution)
Azathioprine (oral suspension)
Baclofen (oral suspension)
Bethanechol (oral suspension, oral solution)
BPND mouthwash (oral liquid)

Busulfan (oral suspension)
Caffeine (injection, oral solution)
Calcitriol (oral liquid)
Captopril (oral solution)
Carbamazepine (oral suspension)
Carboxymethylcellulose Sodium (oral suspension)
Carisoprodol (oral suspension)
Carvedilol (oral suspension)
Cefazolin (ophthalmic drops)
Cefuroxime (ophthalmic drops)
Chlorambucil (oral suspension)
Chloroquine (oral suspension)
Chlorothiazide (oral suspension)
Cholesterol (oral suspension)
Cholestyramine/Petrolatum (topical ointment)
Cimetidine Hydrochloride (injection, oral suspension)
Ciprofloxacin (oral suspension)
Cisapride (oral suspension)
Clindamycin (injection)
Clonazepam (oral suspension)
Clonidine (oral suspension)
Clopidrogel Bisulfate (oral suspension)
Cocaine (topical solution)
Codeine phosphate (oral syrup)
Cortisone Acetate (oral suspension)
Cyclophosphamide (oral suspension, oral elixir)
Cyclosporine (ophthalmic solution, paste)
Dantrolene (oral suspension)
Dapsone (oral suspension)
Desmopressin (intranasal solution)
Dexamethasone sodium phosphate (injection)

Diazepam (oral suspension)
Diazoxide (oral suspension)
Diltiazem (oral suspension, oral solution)
Diphtheria/Tetanus Toxoids, Adsorbed (skin test)
Dipyridamole (oral suspension)
Disopyramide (oral suspension)
Dolasetron Mesylate (oral suspension)
Doxycycline (oral suspension)
Edetate Calcium Disodium with Procaine Hydrochloride (injection)
Enalapril (oral suspension)
Ethacrynic acid (oral solution)
Ethambutol (oral suspension)
Ethanol for catheter clearance (injection)
Ethinyl Estradiol (diluting fluid, compounding solution)
Etoposide (oral solution)
Famotidine (oral suspension)
Fentanyl (nasal solution)
Flecainide (oral suspension)
Fluconazole (oral liquid)
Flucytosine (oral suspension)
Fluoxetine (oral solution)
Folic Acid (oral solution)
Fumagillin (ophthalmic solution)
Furosemide (oral liquid)
Gabapentin (oral suspension)
Ganciclovir (oral suspension)
Gentamicin Sulfate, Fortified (ophthalmic drops)
Glutamine (oral suspension)
Glycine (aminoacetic acid) (oral solution)
Glycopyrrolate (oral suspension)
Granisetron (oral suspension)

Griseofulvin (oral suspension)
Hydralazine (injection, oral solution, oral suspension)
Hydrochloric Acid 0.1 Normal (catheter clearance injection)
Hydrochlorothiazide (oral suspension)
Hydrocortisone (oral suspension)
Hydrocortisone sodium phosphate (injection)
Hydrocortisone/Neomycin (enema)
Hydroquinone (ointment)
Hydroxychloroquine (oral suspension)
Hydroxypropylmethylcellulose (oral suspension)
Hydroxyurea (oral solution)
Indomethacin (oral suspension)
Isoniazid (oral suspension)
Isradipine (oral suspension)
Itraconazole (oral suspension)
Ketoconazole (oral suspension)
Labetalol (oral suspension)
Lamotrigine (oral suspension)
Lansoprazole (oral suspension)
Levodopa/carbidopa (oral suspension)
Levofloxacin (oral suspension)
Levothyroxine (oral suspension)
Lidocaine, Epinephrine, and Tetracaine, topical (solution, gel)
Lisinopril (oral suspension)
Lorazepam (oral suspension, injection)
Losartan (oral suspension)
Mercaptopurine (oral suspension)
MESNA (oral solution)
Methotrexate (oral suspension)
Methylcellulose (oral suspension)
Methyldopa (oral suspension, oral solution)

Methylphenidate (oral suspension)
Methylprednisolone Sodium Succinate (injection)
Metolazone (oral suspension)
Metoprolol (oral suspension)
Metronidazole (oral suspension)
Metronidazole/Ceftizoxime (injection)
Mexiletine (oral suspension)
Midazolam (oral solution, flavored gelatin)
Mitomycin (ophthalmic drops)
Morphine (oral solution, injection)
Moxifloxacin (oral suspension)
Mupirocin (topical ointment)
Mycophenolate (oral suspension)
Nadolol (oral suspension)
Naratriptan (oral suspension)
Nifedipine (oral suspension, oral solution)
Nizatidine (oral suspension)
Norfloxacin (oral suspension)
Omeprazole (oral suspension)
Ondansetron (oral suspension)
Oral preoperative sedative (oral solution)
Oseltamivir (oral suspension)
Penicillamine (oral suspension)
Pentoxifylline (oral suspension)
Phenobarbital (injection, oral suspension, oral solution)
Phenoxybenzamine (oral solution)
Phytonadione (oral suspension, oral solution)
Pilocarpine (oral solution)
Potassium Perchlorate (oral syrup)
Pravastatin (oral suspension)
Prednisolone (oral solution)

Prednisone (oral solution)
Primaquine (oral suspension)
Procainamide (oral suspension)
Procaine Hydrochloride (injection)
Procarbazine Hydrochloride (oral powder)
Propranolol (oral solution)
Propylthiouracil (oral suspension)
Pyrazinamide (oral suspension)
Pyridoxine Hydrochloride (oral solution)
Pyrimethamine (oral suspension)
Quinapril Hydrochloride (oral suspension)
Quinidine (oral suspension)
Ranitidine (injection, oral suspension)
Rifabutin (oral suspension)
Rifampin (oral suspension)
Rifaximin (oral suspension)
Rufinamide (oral suspension)
Shohl's solution (oral solution)
Sildenafil (oral suspension)
Sodium Bicarbonate (oral solution)
Sodium Hypochlorite (topical solution)
Sodium Phenylbutyrate (oral suspension)
Sotalol (oral suspension)
Spironolactone (oral suspension)
Spironolactone/Hydrochlorothiazide (oral suspension)
Sucralfate (oral suspension)
Sumatriptan (oral suspension)
Sunitinib (oral suspension)
Tacrolimus (oral suspension)
Terbinafine Hydrochloride (oral suspension)

Terbutaline (oral suspension)
Tetracycline (oral suspension, ophthalmic ointment)
Thioguanine (oral suspension)
Three Bromides Syrup (oral syrup)
Tiagabine (oral suspension)
Tobramycin (ophthalmic drops)
Topiramate (oral suspension)
Trimethoprim (oral suspension)
Ursodiol (oral suspension)
Valacyclovir (oral suspension)
Verapamil (oral suspension)
Voriconazole (oral suspension)
Zinc Acetate (oral syrup)
Zonisamide (oral suspension)

Preface to the Sixth Edition

We are happy to complete this 6th edition of our book, which continues to be widely used in the US and abroad. This edition contains a total of 363 formulations for use primarily in pediatric patients, although some adults, especially the elderly, may also benefit from their use if they have difficulty swallowing tablets or capsules.

We have added 83 formulations to this edition. As in previous editions, multiple formulations with different vehicles have been included for certain drugs because of varying availability of vehicles in different practice settings in the US and other countries. Some ready-to-use vehicles, like Ora-Plus, Ora-Sweet, Ora-Blend, and SyrSpend, are readily available in the US, but not in many other countries. In that situation, an extemporaneously prepared methylcellulose 1% suspension may be used with syrup in place of the ready-to-use vehicles. Ready-to-use Hypromellose or SnoTears are available in certain countries, but not in the US.

Many drugs used in the pediatric patient have not been approved by the US Food and Drug Administration (FDA) for use in infants and children. When a drug is not approved for use in infants, it is unlikely to be commercially available in a suitable formulation for this population. In a survey of 57 large and small hospitals, we found the need for over 100 stable extemporaneous liquid formulations.[1] Another survey of 20 pediatric hospitals noted that compounded liquid formulations were used for 28% of the inpatients.[2]

The Best Pharmaceuticals for Children Act offers a 6-month marketing exclusivity incentive to the manufacturers of the marketed products that conduct pediatric studies in response to a written request from the FDA. However, this applies to drugs under patents and may be an attractive incentive mainly for commonly used products.

The Pediatric Research Equity Act gives the FDA authority to require pediatric studies if meaningful therapeutic benefit exists. These regulations are positive developments for labeling of medications for use in pediatric patients; however, their impact on the availability of suitable formulations of most generic drugs used in this population has been extremely limited.

Some drugs, such as spironolactone, are available in a liquid formulation abroad but not in the US; the reverse is true for other drugs. If a suitable formulation is available in one country, such should be the case in all countries.

Access to suitable formulations is essential for the proper use of medications in infants and children. Thus, every effort should be made to market the needed formulations. If it is not possible, at least the procedure to prepare a stable dosage form should be included in the package information as has been done for a few drugs, including lisinopril and rifampin.

We are grateful to all the practitioners, educators, and researchers for their contributions to patient care. We also appreciate your continued interest in this book and your suggestions to improve it. We look forward to receiving your comments on the Feedback Forms provided at the back of this book.

Milap C. Nahata
Vinita B. Pai
November 2010

Reference
1. Pai V, Nahata MC. Need for extemporaneous formulations in pediatric patients. J Pediatr Pharmacol Ther 2001;6:107-19.
2. Lugo R, Cash J, Trimby R, Ward R, Spielberg S. A survey of children's hospitals on the use of extemporaneous liquid formulations in the inpatient setting (abstract). J Pediatr Pharmacol Ther 2009;14:156.

Preface to the Fifth Edition

We continue to be pleased with the wide use of this book for preparing extemporaneous drug formulations within the US as well as abroad. A total of 280 extemporaneous formulations are provided for potential use in infants and children. Formulations have been added to this edition. Although these formulations are primarily used in pediatric patients, some have also been used in adults who have difficulty in swallowing tablets or capsules, such as elderly patients or those with dysphagia.

Considering the worldwide need, we have provided multiple formulations of certain drugs. Some ready-to-use vehicles like Ora-Plus or Ora-Sweet are readily available in the US, but not in many other countries. In that situation, an extemporaneously prepared methylcellulose 1% suspension with syrup may be used in place of Ora-Plus and Ora-Sweet. Ready-to-use Hypromellose or SnoTears are available in certain countries, but not in the US.

The need for extemporaneous formulations continues to exist. A recent survey[1] of hospital pharmacists serving pediatric populations found that 76 drug formulations had adequate drug stability information. However, additional stability data were required for 109 drug formulations, and no stability data were available for an additional 103 medications used in infants and young children.

We appreciate your interest in this book and your suggestions to improve it. We look forward to receiving your comments about this publication as well (see page 307 for Feedback Form).

Milap C. Nahata
Vinita B. Pai
Thomas F. Hipple
March 2003

Reference
1. Pai V, Nahata MC. Need for extemporaneous formulations in pediatric patients. J Pediatr Pharmacol Ther 2001;6:107-19.

Preface to the Fourth Edition

Extemporaneous drug formulations continue to play an important role in the treatment of infants and young children. We are pleased to offer this fourth edition, which contains 124 extemporaneous formulations for potential use in pediatric patients. Twenty-seven formulations have been added to this edition.

The majority of drugs approved by the Food and Drug Administration (FDA) have little or no data about their use in infants and children. New FDA regulations may require manufacturers to conduct pediatric studies and seek labeling for new drugs in children. However, this requirement can be waived for a number of reasons, including the difficulty in developing a pediatric formulation, as long as "reasonable efforts" were made. We hope the new regulations will be enforced with a clear definition of "reasonable efforts." Perhaps the most encouraging development is the incentive offered to the industry for pediatric labeling. The FDA would provide a six-month extension of exclusivity and waiver of fees for the supplemental new drug application for pediatric drug development. This may increase labeling of drugs, and thus availability of suitable formulations of new drugs. However, extemporaneous formulations would continue to be necessary for generic drugs, new drugs of little interest to the sponsor, or those infrequently used in children.

We wish to congratulate all pharmacists, physicians, nurses, and technical personnel for their efforts in making medicines accessible to pediatric patients; and researchers for conducting research and sharing data on pediatric drug formulations. We look forward to your comments and suggestions for further improvement of this publication.

Milap C. Nahata
Thomas F. Hipple
May 2000

Preface to the Third Edition

The need for this third edition reflects a continued interest of practitioners, educators, and researchers in pediatric drug formulations. We are happy to be in a position to contribute toward improving the health and well being of pediatric patients. It is good to know that some of the liquid formulations are also being used to treat geriatric patients who experience difficulty in swallowing tablets or capsules.

This edition contains 106 formulations. We have added 35 new formulations. These are suspensions of acetazolamide, allopurinol, amlodipine, azathioprine, cisapride, diltiazem, fluconazole, flucytosine, fluoxetine, gabapentin, granisetron, isradipine, itraconazole, ketoconazole, labetalol, lamotrigine, lorazepam, metoprolol, metronidazole, ondansetron, pentoxifylline, procainamide, procainamide oral liquid, pyrazinamide, ranitidine, spironolactone, spironolactone/hydrochlorothiazide, three bromides syrup, ursodiol, and verapamil. Of the 106 formulations, a specific reference was available for 84 formulations, and clinical experience was cited for 22 formulations. This is improved in comparison with the first two editions of the book. However, new drugs without suitable dosage formulations will continue to be marketed as we complete research on existing drugs.

It is gratifying to observe the progress being made in the area of pediatric pharmacotherapy. It is of great concern, however, that most medications are marketed without adequate studies in and availability of appropriate dosages for infants and children. This trend is likely to continue due to declining resources. We hope that all individuals associated with pediatric pharmacotherapy will take greater responsibility for conducting research and sharing information about pediatric dosage forms.

Milap C. Nahata
Thomas F. Hipple
June 1997

Preface to the Second Edition

We are pleased with the acceptance of our first edition, which was published in 1990. This second edition includes compounding instructions for all formulas, new formulations, revision of existing formulations, and available references for documented stability. We have added 12 new formulas, revised seven formulas, and deleted eight formulas. The new formulas added are amiodarone suspension, captopril solution, dapsone suspension, 70% ethanol injection, flecainide suspension, flucytosine suspension, hydrochloric acid injection, isoniazid suspension, mexiletine suspension, phytonadione suspension, verapamil suspension, and zinc acetate solution. Changes were made to the formulas for acetazolamide suspension, allopurinol suspension, azathioprine suspension, mercaptopurine suspension, morphine injection, oral preoperative sedative, and potassium perchlorate syrup. The formulas deleted are atropine solution, cath mixture injection, disulfiram suspension, lorazepam injection, methyldopate suspension, penicillin V potassium oral powder, sodium hypochlorite, and sodium polystyrene.

This edition of our book covers 71 formulations for administration by intravenous, oral, and rectal routes. In the 37 cases where a specific reference on the stability of a drug is lacking, we have cited our clinical experience as the basis for including the formulation. Unfortunately, the need for these formulations in infants and children cannot wait for definitive stability studies. The fact that nearly one-half of the formulations have no published stability data emphasizes an immediate need for research. A more recent study documented the need for additional information on the compounding and stability of extemporaneous drug formulations.[1]

With a combined total of 45 years of clinical experience in pediatric drug therapy, we continue to find a challenge in meeting the diverse therapeutic needs of pediatric patients. It is our hope that this effort will contribute to optimizing the care of infants and children, and stimulate our future colleagues to actively pursue careers in pediatric pharmacy practice, education, and research.

Milap C. Nahata
Thomas F. Hipple
September 1992

Reference
1. Crawford SY, Dombrowski SR. Extemporaneous compounding activities and the associated informational needs of pharmacists. Am J Hosp Pharm 1991;48:1205-10.

Preface to the First Edition

The needs of drug therapy for infants and children are quite diverse. Although a majority of marketed drugs are used in pediatric patients, only one-fourth of the drugs approved by the Food and Drug Administration have specific indications for use in this population. Those drugs not specifically approved for infants and children are often not available in suitable dosage forms. Even drugs like phenobarbital, aminophylline, and spironolactone, which have been approved for pediatric patients, are not available in the appropriate formulations. Pharmacists are encouraged to prepare extemporaneous drug formulations, make different concentrations or combinations from marketed intravenous drugs, and prepare oral liquid or powder formulations from solid dosage forms (tablets and capsules). Large errors in the measurement of concentrated drugs have caused intoxication with digoxin[1] and morphine[2] in infants. Furthermore, any modification or reformulation of an original drug product raises the question of stability. It is obvious that effective and safe therapy dictates accurate drug administration.

Pediatric pharmacy practitioners either individually or collectively have traditionally sought the assistance of the pharmaceutical industry in relieving the hospital pharmacy of the burden and uncertainty of determining the potency of extemporaneously prepared pediatric dosage forms. Several buying groups as well as the specialty practice group on pediatrics of the American Society of Hospital Pharmacists (ASHP) are currently asking pharmaceutical manufacturers to assist with these problems. The expectations are that the industry will develop and market good-tasting stable dosage forms that will eliminate the need for compounding in pharmacy. However, we must ask the question: Is this a realistic expectation?

Many existing drugs are intrinsically unstable in any aqueous vehicle, assuming that this is the only acceptable vehicle for pediatric oral administration. The limitation of even one year's stability would force the manufacturer to use special distribution systems, because delays in the normal distribution channels would severely limit the shelf life of the drugs.

In considering the size of the pediatric healthcare market as a proportion of the total healthcare market, we must realize that from a business perspective the development of a special pediatric dosage form may be a negative financial venture. With the advent of group purchasing and the general pressure to reduce costs and remove the economic profit from competitive pharmaceuticals, it is not realistic to expect the manufacturer to be at a competitive disadvantage in order to solve our compounding problems. It would seem that the pharmaceutical manufacturer could best help by contributing through the Pharmaceutical Manufacturer's Association Foundation to researchers who can develop basic formulas, determine the stability of drug in each formula, and disseminate that information to pediatric pharmacy practitioners.

The efforts of the ASHP should be commended. At its first meeting in 1975, the Special Interest Group on Pediatric Pharmacy Practice discussed the problems associated with the stability of extemporaneously compounded pediatric dosage forms. A subcommittee of the Special Interest Group was formed in 1977 to gather information on extemporaneous compounding activities in hospitals. The goals of the subcommittee were (1) to collect available information on extemporaneously compounded preparations used in pediatric pharmacy practice that had either documented stability or efficacy; (2) to identify products for which a dosage form was not available and yet which might be of use in pediatric practice; (3) to disseminate the information obtained to pharmacy practitioners; and (4) to encourage and pursue research efforts for new formulations and testing of existing essential products used in pediatric practice that had only suggested or unproven efficacy.

The "Report of the Subcommittee on Pediatric Extemporaneous Formulations" by the ASHP Special Interest Group on Pediatric Pharmacy Practice was published in 1979. That publication used three categories to identify drug stability data. A designation of class I meant that published information on stability existed and references were cited. Class II indicated that the pharmacist submitting the formula had communicated with the manufacturer about the stability. A class III designation indicated only personal experience. The published list had eight formulas categorized as class I, 22 as class II, and 22 as class

III. Illustrating the lack of progress made since then, the ASHP *Handbook on Extemporaneous Formulations* published in 1987 cites no references on stability for 23 of 51 formulations.[3]

There are three major limitations of the ASHP *Handbook:* (1) it provides formulations only for oral suspensions and liquids; (2) a number of formulations contain methylcellulose 9% (Cologel, Lilly), which is very thick and thus difficult to work with and is no longer available commercially in the US; and (3) a stability period is indicated for certain formulations but no specific references are cited. Stability information without references signifies that it originated from the individual contributing pharmacists based on their experience. Stability may thus be difficult to ascertain because different institutions could have different criteria for establishing stability and varying degrees of clinical experience with a given formulation.

A similar compilation, *Extemporaneous Oral Liquid Dosage Preparations,* published in 1988 by the Canadian Society of Hospital Pharmacists, categorized drug stability as class I when published data were on file and as class II when stability was assumed but no data were available. It is important to note that 91 of 130 formulations were listed under class II.[4]

We wrote this book because there is a clear need for a publication on extemporaneous formulations for infants and children. No other book contains a variety of extemporaneous formulations for intravenous and oral use with documented stability data and years of experience.

Although a variety of healthcare professionals other than pharmacists (e.g., nurses and physicians) may find the information contained here to be useful, it should be particularly useful in (1) departments of pharmacy in pediatric institutions as well as hospitals at-large serving neonatal or pediatric patients; (2) libraries in colleges of pharmacy and health sciences; and (3) community pharmacies receiving prescriptions that must be extemporaneously compounded for pediatric use. A significant number of patients can benefit from this information.

Milap C. Nahata
Thomas F. Hipple
March 1990

References
1. Berman W, Whitman V, Marks KH, Friedman Z, Maisal MJ, Musselman J. Inadvertent overadministration of digoxin to low birth weight infants. J Pediatr 1978;

92:1024-5.
2. Zenk KE, Anderson S. Improving the accuracy of mini-volume injections. Infusion 1982;6:7-11.
3. Committee on Extemporaneous Formulations, Special Interest Group on Pediatric Pharmacy Practice. Handbook on extemporaneous formulations. Bethesda, MD: American Society of Hospital Pharmacists, 1987:1-54.
4. McCrea J, Rappaport P, Stansfield S, Baker D, Dupuis LL, James G. Extemporaneous oral liquid dosage preparations. Toronto: Canadian Society of Hospital Pharmacists, 1988:1-24.

Introduction to the Formulations

With so few approved drugs available in dosage forms appropriate for infants and children, compounding extemporaneous formulation is a significant portion of pharmacists' work in many pediatric settings. Generally, tablets and capsules are converted to oral liquid (suspensions) or powder forms. Intravenous drugs are sometimes administered orally, and intravenous or oral preparations are used rectally.

An ideal formulation should (1) be easily prepared by a pharmacist and administered by a nurse, (2) have appropriate drug concentration and volume for accurate administration, (3) be palatable to ensure patient compliance, and (4) have documented drug stability data. Intravenous dosage forms that are not commercially available should be tested for sterility, pyrogens, and stability in accordance with the *United States Pharmacopeia* (USP) and the *National Formulary* (NF) standards.

Concentrated intravenous drugs intended for adults (e.g., digoxin, morphine, phenobarbital) may have to be diluted in appropriate vehicles for use in children. For example, phenobarbital is available at a concentration of 65 mg/mL, but volumes as low as 0.01 mL may have to be measured to provide the recommend dose for infants. To accomplish this, we dilute phenobarbital in sodium chloride 0.9% injection to achieve a concentration of 10 mg/mL. Because the original product contains propylene glycol to improve stability, it may seem logical to dilute it with propylene glycol. However, because propylene glycol has been found to cause hyperosmolality in infants,[1] further addition of that vehicle would not be wise. When an original formulation is altered in any way, the stability of the drug must be documented. We showed[2] that phenobarbital was stable in the reformulated product before initiating its use in patients.

Intravenous drugs such as methyldopa and bethanechol are used orally in infants and children. Tablets of many drugs, such as acetazolamide and spironolactone, are crushed to prepare suspensions. Rifampin capsules are used to make its liquid dosage form. Oral liquids (e.g., acetaminophen pediatric drops) have been used rectally in newborn infants. Each of these modifications requires either preparation immediately before administering each dose or proof of stability of the drug in a reformulated preparation. The manufacturers can usually provide the stability data only for their original product, which is of little help to clinicians needing data on the new formulation. Moreover, few departments of pharmacy are equipped to conduct research on the chemical stability of drugs using stability-indicating analytical methods. We believe the scarcity of stability data limits a wide use of optimally reformulated drugs in infants and children.

Considerations for Preparing Extemporaneous Compounds

The ability of the vehicle to suspend the powdered active ingredients is of primary importance to the quality of the suspensions. Some suspending agents allow the particles to settle and form a compact sediment at the bottom of the container, requiring prolonged shaking to reconstitute a uniform suspension. If dispensed into unit-dose containers, will the preparations be shaken adequately by nursing personnel administering the medications? How will the suspension be stored and used when sent home with the patient?

Methylcellulose or methylcellulose/syrup combination can be considered as a nearly universal suspending agent for pediatric liquid preparations. These ingredients are almost as inert, nonreactive, and pH-neutral as any agent available, with the possible exception of water, which is not a suspending agent.

The preparation of methylcellulose solution is difficult. Some publications[3] recommend a procedure that requires the use of a blender and nearly 4 hours to clear the bubbles. Our experience has shown that we often need to use the methylcellulose solution before 4 hours have passed. Therefore, we have developed a procedure whereby the methylcellulose powder is mixed with alcohol (5% of total volume) to make a slurry, which is then added to rapidly stirred cold water. The resulting preparation is cloudy; however, it is uniform in content and can be used immediately. We have found that using a blender to mix methylcellulose causes so much air entrapment that measuring the proper final volume is impossible for several days.

For the above reasons, it is generally desirable to have the suspending vehicle prepared and ready to use so that preparation of the suspension can proceed as soon as the need is recognized. We use alcohol 5% when compounding methylcellulose and carboxymethylcellulose suspending agents to retard the growth of microorganisms.

Carboxymethylcellulose sodium is easier to work with than methylcellulose, but it has a pH of approximately 10. Use of this material as a suspending agent could result in a reaction with acidic drugs and potentially change important characteristics of these drugs.

Most pharmacists in the US may prefer to incorporate ready-to-use Ora-Plus as a suspending agent and Ora-Sweet as a syrup with or without sugar in 1:1 volume. These vehicles have been widely used in conducting stability studies and are suitable for most drugs. The pH of Ora-Plus is 4.2, which should be considered in compounding suspensions when drug stability data are unavailable for the preparation. Ora-Blend is now available ready-to-use in a 1:1 proportion of Ora-Plus and Ora-Sweet; this is also available in a sugar-free form as Ora-Blend SF (Paddock Lab, Minneapolis, MN). This avoids the need to mix 2 ready-to-use vehicles into 1 vehicle. Additional commercially available vehicles include SyrSpend and SyrSpend SF (Alka, Cherry, Alka Cherry, Grape, and Alka Grape) as ready-to-use suspending agents with syrup (Gallipot Inc., St. Paul, MN).

The formulations in this book have listed the type of syrup that we originally used in preparing the extemporaneous dosage form. Special flavoring agents are not universally available in standardized products. In such cases, appropriate flavor additions can be made within each institution according to its individual needs. Numerous flavors are available from FlavoRx (Columbia, MD) for use in formulations, although we have not used these in our patients or to conduct stability studies. Simple syrup, NF (85% sucrose in water) is a standardized product without preservatives and can be used in place of flavored syrups without affecting the stability of active ingredients. Some formulations recommend the use of wild cherry syrup. Some wild cherry-flavored syrups may be satisfactory vehicles, but wild cherry syrup, USP, was formulated as an expectorant and has a bitter taste. If desired, it can be replaced with simple syrup, NF.

Much attention has been given to the dangers of using preservatives in extemporaneously prepared pediatric oral liquids. Equal consideration should be given to the risk involved in distributing extemporaneously prepared suspensions contaminated with microorganisms, especially to the immunocompromised patient. We have observed that air contamination of a methylcellulose syrup mixture can result in the growth of molds unless a preservative is added. Preservatives used in appropriate concentrations in extemporaneous preparations may not present any more danger to the patient than that associated with administration of commercially prepared preserved drugs. To minimize microbial growth, we recommend refrigeration for storage. When available, the stability data at room temperature have been included to assess the potency of drugs if the bottles had to be stored at room temperature due to lack of availability of a refrigerator, such as during travel or when inadvertently left outside the refrigerator for brief periods. Although most stability studies have been done at 22–25 °C, the room temperature can range from

40 °C to 50 °C and refrigerators may not be available for storage of medications in certain countries. The impact of such conditions on drug stability is often unknown.

When stability data are lacking, it has been suggested that tablets can be crushed by nurses just prior to drug administration and children can be taught to swallow oral medications.[4] It may often be impractical to divide a 5-mg tablet to provide a 1-mg dose. Furthermore, the preparation of the drug dosage form should be a pharmacist's responsibility, not a nurse's. Although some children can be taught to swallow oral solid dosage forms, those younger than five years of age often cannot. The osmolality of suspensions and syrup has also been suggested as a cause for concern.[4] Theoretically this may be true, but the osmolality of most suspensions and syrups contributes a small fraction of the osmolality of oral feedings most patients would receive.

The 280 formulations described in this book include ophthalmic oral, rectal, and injectable products. Specific references on drug stability for similar formulations have been cited when available. The formulations are listed alphabetically based on the generic names of the primary drugs or the common names of certain much-used formulations.

The formulas list the USP grade ingredients, amounts, and instructions for preparation. We have made a general assumption that a pharmacist will use this information as a guideline for the actual preparation of the compounds according to generally accepted compounding practices. We have not provided general compounding instructions; therefore, remarks in the "Instructions" sections should be considered special requirements of the particular formula. For formulations without instructions in the original source, we have provided a method, but individual[5] practitioners may prefer their own compounding procedures.

Some formulas described in the cited literature have used Cologel (Lilly) as a suspending agent. This product, which was a flavored concentrated methylcellulose suspension, has been discontinued by the manufacturer. We have substituted our methylcellulose preparation for Cologel in these formulations. An additional source of flavored methylcellulose suspending agent is described in the pyrazinamide formula. Citrucel (Aventis) is an over-the-counter bulk laxative preparation commonly found in community pharmacies. A flavored methylcellulose 1% suspending vehicle can be made by adding 25.5 g to 500 mL of water.

Patient acceptance of a liquid dosage form is largely dependent on its palatability. A better-tasting drug would be easier to administer to infants and young children, and thus minimize loss of drug from spillage during dose administration. In general, compliance may be enhanced with improved taste.

The taste of drug formulations should be evaluated in children by using a five-point hedonic (facial expression) scale.[5] The overall taste perception should reflect initial taste, aftertaste, flavor, and texture of the formulation. Interestingly, taste is rarely studied in children, even for commercially available formulations; these studies are generally done in adults. It is difficult to predict whether the Human Subjects Research Committee would approve such comparative studies in children.

There are 3 types of information in the "Stability Reference" sections. A number signifies a citation in a reference listing, referring to a report published in the literature. Storage temperature between 4 and 5 °C refers to refrigerated temperature and that ranging from 22 to 25 °C is considered room temperature. The storage container is generally an amber plastic prescription bottle and is usually preferred; containers are specifically indicated as used in studies. We have also clearly mentioned whether a stability-indicating method was not used by authors cited in the references in conducting stability studies. Similarly, we have mentioned whether sterility and pyrogen testing was not done by researchers for intravenously administered extemporaneous formulations. In some cases, authors cited may have concluded a drug to be stable at 90 ± 3% of the initial concentration, but we have not done so in this book since the lowest concentration could be 87% of the original concentration, when considering the standard deviation. "Experience" refers to our experience in compounding the formulation. In some cases, we have obtained stability information from a drug manufacturer or another healthcare institution; these are listed as "personal communication" and followed by the source's name and date of communication.

We have included some commercially available formulations for 2 reasons. First, the drug concentration of a commercially available product may limit its use. Second, drug shortage for commercial products may occur on certain occasions.

All commercially available and extemporaneously prepared formulations contain therapeutically inactive ingredients (excipients) to serve various functions, such as diluents, wetting agents, solvents, binders, fillers, preservatives, sweeteners, and stabilizing, coloring, or flavoring agents.[6] Although these are generally considered inert, their safety cannot be assumed. For example, the Food and Drug Administration has recommended exclusion of benzyl alcohol for newborns due to serious toxicities including metabolic acidosis, respiratory and central nervous system depression, and death.[7,8]

Acceptable daily intakes of excipients have been suggested by the World Health Organization for adults, but such information is unknown for the pediatric population. Infants and children are exposed to a variety of excipients, such as benzyl alcohol, ethanol, propylene glycol, and sorbitol present in the medications, so the safety of cumulative exposure needs to be determined. Excipients are listed by name on the label, but the amounts of most excipients are not: the amounts should be listed so that practitioners can consider their safety in patients. Critically ill patients receiving continuous infusions of medications are likely to be exposed to the highest amounts of excipients per day and premature infants are most likely to have the lowest clearance of excipients; thus, these populations should be monitored for safe use of excipients.[6]

Following the formulation section, 5 pages have been included so that you can add your own formulations to the book. The Feedback Form on page 307 is our way of encouraging you to send us formulations or comments regarding the formulations published here.

Finally, we urge that practitioners use their clinical judgment when recommending extemporaneous formulations for their patients. Physical and chemical stability may not guarantee bioavailability, bioequivalence, or safety. Practitioners should monitor for the efficacy and safety of extemporaneous formulations.

References
1. Glasgow AM, Boerckx RL, Miller MK, MacDonald MG, August GP, Goodman SI. Hyperosmolality in small infants due to propylene glycol. Pediatrics 1983; 72:353-5.
2. Nahata MC, Hipple TF, Strausbaugh S. Stability of phenobarbital sodium diluted in 0.9% NaCl for injection. Am J Hosp Pharm 1986;43:384-5.
3. McCrea J, Rappaport P, Stansfield S, Baker D, Dupuis LL, James G. Extemporaneous oral liquid dosage preparations. Toronto: Canadian Society of Hospital Pharmacists, 1988:1-24.
4. Committee on Extemporaneous Formulations, Special Interest Group on Pediatric Pharmacy Practice. Handbook on extemporaneous formulations. Bethesda, MD: American Society of Hospital Pharmacists, 1987:1-54.
5. Matsui D, Barron A, Rieder MJ. Assessment of the palatability of antistaphylococcal antibiotics in pediatric volunteers. Ann Pharmacother 1996;30:586-8.
6. Nahata MC. Safety of "inert" additives or excipients in paediatric medicines. Arch Dis Child Fetal Neonatal Ed 2009;94:392-3.
7. Lopez-Herce J, Bonet C, Meana A, Albajara L. Benzyl alcohol poisoning following diazepam intravenous infusion (letter). Ann Pharmacother 1995;29:632.
8. Gershanik J, Boecler B, Ensley H, et al. The gasping syndrome and benzyl alcohol poisoning. N Engl J Med 1982;307:1384-8.

GENERIC NAME	**Acetazolamide**
DOSAGE FORM	oral suspension
MADE FROM	tablets
CONCENTRATION	25 mg/mL
STABILITY	60 days
STABILITY REFERENCE	Allen LV Jr, et al. Am J Health Syst Pharm 1996; 53:1944-9
STORE	refrigerate (preferable) or at room temperature
LABEL	shake well before use, refrigerate

INGREDIENT	STRENGTH	QUANTITY
Acetazolamide tablets	250 mg	12
Cherry syrup concentrate (diluted 1:4 with simple syrup, NF)		qs 120 mL

INSTRUCTIONS: Crush the tablets and triturate to a fine powder. Add approximately 20 mL of vehicle and levigate to a uniform paste. Add vehicle in geometric proportions almost to volume, mix thoroughly, and transfer to a graduate. Rinse the mortar with vehicle, add to the graduate, and qs to 120 mL.

NOTES

GENERIC NAME	**Acetazolamide**
DOSAGE FORM	oral suspension
MADE FROM	tablets
CONCENTRATION	25 mg/mL
STABILITY	79 days
STABILITY REFERENCE	Alexander KS, et al. Am J Hosp Pharm 1991; 48:1241-4
STORE	refrigerate (preferable) or room temperature
LABEL	shake well before use, refrigerate, protect from light

INGREDIENT	STRENGTH	QUANTITY
Acetazolamide tablets	250 mg	30
Sorbitol solution	70%	30 mL
Carboxymethylcellulose sodium		1.5 g
Purified water, NF		qs 300 mL
Aluminum magnesium silicate		1.5 g
Simple syrup USP		60 mL
Glycerine USP		7.5 mL
Paraben stock solution		6 mL
FD&C red no. 40		0.015 g
Strawberry flavor		0.3 mL
Hydrochloric acid	36% w/w	qs to adjust pH to 4-5

NOTE: In this study, the formulation was stored in amber glass bottles and maintained at pH 4-5.

INSTRUCTIONS: Crush the acetazolamide tablets into a fine powder in a glass mortar. Levigate the powder by adding 70% sorbitol solution into a smooth paste. In a beaker, hydrate carboxymethylcellulose sodium for 15-20 minutes by slowly adding it to 50 mL of warm purified water. In another beaker, add aluminum magnesium silicate to another 50 mL of purified water. Combine the hydrated carboxymethylcellulose and dispersed aluminum magnesium silicate with the levigated powder in geometric proportions with constant mixing. To this, geometrically incorporate simple syrup, glycerin, and the paraben stock solution, with constant stirring to produce a homogenous mixture. (The paraben stock solution is prepared by dissolving 0.25 g of methylparaben and 0.1 g of propylparaben in 10 mL of propylene glycol.) Transfer the acetazolamide mixture to a graduate. Add the coloring and flavoring agent. Rinse the mortar with 30-mL portions of purified water and transfer to the graduate. Repeat the steps to make the final volume 300 mL. Homogenize using a suitable blender. Adjust the pH of the mixture to 5, using hydrochloric acid.

NOTES

GENERIC NAME	**Acetazolamide**
DOSAGE FORM	oral suspension
MADE FROM	tablets
CONCENTRATION	25 mg/mL
STABILITY	60 days (5 °C and 25 °C)
STABILITY REFERENCE	Allen LV Jr, et al. Am J Health Syst Pharm 1996; 53:1944-9
STORE	refrigerate (preferable) or at room temperature
LABEL	shake well before use, refrigerate

INGREDIENT	STRENGTH	QUANTITY
Acetazolamide tablets	250 mg	12
Ora-Plus:Ora-Sweet	1:1	
or Ora-Plus:Ora-Sweet SF		qs 120 mL

NOTE: In this study, the formulation was stored in amber clear plastic (polyethylene terephthalate) prescription ovals.

INSTRUCTIONS: Crush the tablets and triturate to a fine powder. Add approximately 20 mL of vehicle and levigate to a uniform paste. Add vehicle in geometric proportions almost to volume and mix thoroughly. Transfer to a graduate and qs to volume with vehicle. Mix well.

NOTES

GENERIC NAME	**Acetazolamide**
DOSAGE FORM	oral suspension
MADE FROM	tablets
CONCENTRATION	25 mg/mL
STABILITY	79 days
STABILITY REFERENCE	experience
STORE	use amber-colored glass bottles, refrigerate
LABEL	shake well before use, refrigerate

INGREDIENT	STRENGTH	QUANTITY
Acetazolamide tablets	250 mg	100
Methylcellulose	1%	300 mL
Veegum		10 g
Syrup		300 mL
[a]Parabens concentration		10 mL
Flavor/purified water, USP		qs 1000 mL

[a]Methylparaben 120 mg, propylparaben 12 mg, propylene glycol qs ad 100 mL.

INSTRUCTIONS: Add the Veegum to 200 mL of water in a blender and blend until uniform. Place the Veegum, methylcellulose, and syrup into a 1-L graduate and mix well. Place the acetazolamide tablets into a blender with 100 mL of water and blend until uniform. Add the blended tablets to the Veegum/methylcellulose syrup mixture. Rinse blender well with water and qs with water, flavoring, and paraben concentrate. You may choose to powder the tablets with a mortar and pestle rather than using a blender.

NOTES

GENERIC NAME	**Acetazolamide**
DOSAGE FORM	oral solution
MADE FROM	tablet
CONCENTRATION	5 mg/mL
STABILITY	178 days at 25 °C and 37 °C
STABILITY REFERENCE	Parasrampuria J, Das Gupta V. J Pharm Sci. 1990;79:835-6
STORE	room temperature
LABEL	shake well before use

INGREDIENT	STRENGTH	QUANTITY
Acetazolamide tablet	500 mg	1
Polyethylene glycol 400		7 mL
Propylene glycol		53 mL
Sorbitol solution (70% w/w)		15 mL
Simple syrup		15 mL
Saccharin sodium		0.18 g
Aspartame		0.18 g
Sodium benzoate		0.2 g
FDC Red #40		58.8 ppm
FDC Blue #1		1.2 ppm
Raspberry flavor		0.05 mL
Sweet flavor		0.3 mL
Menthol		0.002 g
Ethanol		0. 5 mL
Buffer solution (phosphate or citrate in solution)	0.1 M	qs to achieve a pH of 4

NOTE: No information about the type of storage containers is provided in this study.

INSTRUCTIONS: Triturate the tablet into a fine powder. Add polyethylene glycol 400 (PG400) in geometric proportions, with constant mixing to solubilize acetazolamide. To this, add the propylene glycol in geometric proportions, with constant mixing. Dissolve menthol in ethanol and add this solution to the PG400 and propylene glycol mixture. In another container mix the artificial sweeteners, raspberry flavor, and the sweet flavor with simple syrup to which sodium benzoate and sorbitol were added. Mix the simple syrup and PG400 mixture together in geometric proportions. Add the dye solutions to this mixture. Add the buffer solution to adjust the pH of the formulation to 4.

NOTES

GENERIC NAME	**Acetylcysteine**
DOSAGE FORM	oral solution
MADE FROM	solution for inhalation
CONCENTRATION	86.5 mg/mL
STABILITY	35 days
STABILITY REFERENCE	Siden R, et al. Am J Health Syst Pharm 2008;65:558-61
STORE	refrigerate (nontransparent) or room temperature, protect from light
LABEL	shake well before use, refrigerate, protect from light

INGREDIENT	STRENGTH	QUANTITY
Acetylcysteine solution	10%	90 mL
Sweetener FlavoRx		7 mL
Strawberry Creamsicle FlavoRx		7 mL

NOTE: In this study, the formulation was stored in amber prescription bottles.

INSTRUCTIONS: The sweetener and the strawberry creamsicle flavor were added to 90 mL of acetylcysteine solution (10%) in geometric proportions, with constant stirring.

NOTES

Acetylcysteine Ophthalmic Solution

GENERIC NAME	
DOSAGE FORM	ophthalmic solution
MADE FROM	solution
CONCENTRATION	10%
STABILITY	60 days (2–8 °C)
STABILITY REFERENCE	Anaizi NH, et al. Am J Health Syst Pharm 1997; 54:549-53
STORE	refrigerate
LABEL	refrigerate, for ophthalmic use only

INGREDIENT	STRENGTH	QUANTITY
Acetylcysteine solution	20%	7.5 mL
Ophthalmic diluent (chlorbutanol, USP 0.5% in Liquifilm Tears)		7.5 mL

NOTE: Sterility testing not performed.

INSTRUCTIONS: In a mortar, triturate chlorbutanol, USP, and dissolve in approximately 80 mL of artificial tears (Liquifilm Tears). Transfer to a graduate and qs to 100 mL with artificial tears. Pass this solution through a 0.2-μm filter into sterile, pyrogen-free vials in a laminar air flow hood using aseptic technique. This solution is referred to as the ophthalmic diluent. In a sterile 15-mL ophthalmic dropper bottle, mix 7.5 mL of the ophthalmic diluent with 7.5 mL of sterile acetylcysteine 20% solution using sterile syringes and aseptic technique. American Society of Health-System Pharmacists' guidelines (Am J Hosp Pharm 1993;50:1462-3) for compounding ophthalmic products should be considered while preparing this formulation.

NOTES

Acetylcysteine Ophthalmic Solution

GENERIC NAME	Acetylcysteine Ophthalmic Solution
DOSAGE FORM	ophthalmic solution
MADE FROM	solution
CONCENTRATION	10%
STABILITY	90 days (2–8 °C)
STABILITY REFERENCE	Fawcett JP, et al. Aust J Hosp Pharm 1993;23: 18-21
STORE	refrigerate
LABEL	refrigerate, for ophthalmic use only

INGREDIENT	STRENGTH	QUANTITY
Acetylcysteine solution	20%	7.5 mL
Ophthalmic diluent (0.5 mL benzalkonium chloride 0.16% solution added to 7 mL of Isopto Tears)		7.5 mL

NOTE: Sterility testing not performed.

INSTRUCTIONS: Mix benzalkonium solution with the artificial tears (Isopto Tears). Pass this solution through a 0.2-μm filter into sterile, pyrogen-free vials under a laminar air flow hood using aseptic technique. This solution is referred to as the ophthalmic diluent. In a sterile 15-mL ophthalmic dropper bottle, mix 7.5 mL of the ophthalmic diluent with 7.5 mL of sterile acetylcysteine 20% solution using sterile syringes and aseptic technique. American Society of Health-System Pharmacists' guidelines (Am J Hosp Pharm 1993;50:1462-3) for compounding ophthalmic products should be considered while preparing this formulation.

NOTES

Acetylcysteine Ophthalmic Solution

GENERIC NAME	
DOSAGE FORM	ophthalmic solution
MADE FROM	injection
CONCENTRATION	10%
STABILITY	120 days at 2–8 °C; under in-use conditions after 90 days of storage at 2–8 °C, stable for 21 days at 25 °C and 30 days if refrigerated
STABILITY REFERENCE	Fawcett JP, et al. Aust J Hosp Pharm 1993;23: 18-21
STORE	refrigerate, low-density polyethylene eye drop bottles
LABEL	refrigerate, for ophthalmic use only

INGREDIENT	STRENGTH	QUANTITY
N-acetylcysteine injection	20%	7.5 mL
Benzalkonium chloride solution	0.16% w/v	0.5 mL
Isopto Ophthalmic Solution	0.5%	7 mL

NOTE:	Isopto Ophthalmic Solution is a 0.5% hydroxylpropyl methylcellulose containing 0.01% benzalkonium chloride. Additional benzalkonium chloride is added to maintain the same concentration of benzalkonium chloride in the finished product. In this study, the formulation was stored in the sterile Isopto Ophthalmic Solution bottle.
INSTRUCTIONS:	Prepare the eye drops aseptically under appropriate laminar air flood hood. Draw the N-acetylcysteine injection solution, the benzalkonium chloride solution, and the Isopto Ophthalmic Solution into individual sterile syringes. Combine them into a sterile Isopto Ophthalmic Solution bottle by filtering them through a 0.2-μm membrane filter. The pH of the final solution should be 7.3.

NOTES

GENERIC NAME	**Adderall**
DOSAGE FORM	oral suspension
MADE FROM	tablets
CONCENTRATION	1 mg/mL
STABILITY	30 days at room temperature and 60% relative humidity
STABILITY REFERENCE	Justice J, et al. Am J Health Syst Pharm 2001; 58:1418-21
STORE	room temperature
LABEL	shake well before use, protect from light

INGREDIENT	STRENGTH	QUANTITY
Adderall tablets	10 mg	10
Ora-Plus:Ora-Sweet	1:1	qs 100 mL

NOTE: In this study, the formulation was stored in amber glass bottles

INSTRUCTIONS: Mix equal quantities of Ora-Plus and Ora-Sweet in geometric proportions to obtain sufficient quantity of the vehicle. Triturate the tablets into a fine powder in a glass mortar. Add small portion of the vehicle and levigate into a smooth suspension. Add more vehicle, with constant mixing. Transfer the suspension to a graduate. Rinse the mortar with small quantities of the vehicle and transfer to the graduate to make up the final volume.

NOTES

GENERIC NAME	**Allopurinol**
DOSAGE FORM	oral suspension
MADE FROM	tablets
CONCENTRATION	20 mg/mL
STABILITY	60 days
STABILITY REFERENCE	Allen LV Jr, et al. Am J Health Syst Pharm 1996; 53:1944-9
STORE	refrigerate (preferable) or at room temperature
LABEL	shake well before use, refrigerate

INGREDIENT	STRENGTH	QUANTITY
Allopurinol tablets	300 mg	8
Cherry syrup (cherry syrup concentrate diluted 1:4 with simple syrup, NF)		qs 120 mL

NOTE: In this study, the formulation was stored in amber clear plastic (polyethylene terephthalate) prescription ovals.

INSTRUCTIONS: Crush the tablets and triturate to a fine powder. Add approximately 20 mL of vehicle and levigate to a uniform paste. Add vehicle in geometric proportions almost to volume, mix thoroughly, and transfer to a graduate. Rinse the mortar with vehicle, add to the graduate, and qs to 120 mL.

NOTES

GENERIC NAME	**Allopurinol**
DOSAGE FORM	oral suspension
MADE FROM	tablets
CONCENTRATION	20 mg/mL
STABILITY	60 days
STABILITY REFERENCE	Allen LV Jr, et al. Am J Health Syst Pharm 1996; 53:1944-9
STORE	refrigerate (preferable) or at room temperature
LABEL	shake well before use, refrigerate

INGREDIENT	STRENGTH	QUANTITY
Allopurinol tablets	300 mg	8
Ora-Sweet or Ora-Sweet SF		
Ora-Plus		aa qs 120 mL

NOTE: In this study, the formulation was stored in amber clear plastic (polyethylene terephthalate) prescription ovals.

INSTRUCTIONS: Crush the tablets and triturate to a fine powder. Add approximately 20 mL of vehicle and levigate to a uniform paste. Add vehicle in geometric proportions almost to volume, mix thoroughly, and transfer to a graduate. Rinse the mortar with vehicle, add to the graduate, and qs to 120 mL.

NOTES

GENERIC NAME	**Allopurinol**
DOSAGE FORM	oral suspension
MADE FROM	tablets
CONCENTRATION	20 mg/mL
STABILITY	56 days
STABILITY REFERENCE	Dressman JB, et al. Am J Hosp Pharm 1983;40: 616-8
STORE	refrigerate (preferable) or at room temperature
LABEL	shake well before use, refrigerate

INGREDIENT	STRENGTH	QUANTITY
Allopurinol tablet	100 mg	20
Methylcellulose	1%	
Simple syrup, NF		aa qs 100 mL

NOTE: Stability-indicating analytical methods not used. In this study, the formulation contained Cologel 33 mL and wild cherry syrup:simple syrup, NF (1:2) qs 100 mL of 20 mg/mL of the formulation. Cologel, a commercially available vehicle consisting of methylcellulose 9% solution, is no longer available. In the above formulation, Cologel can be substituted with methylcellulose 1% solution and the wild cherry syrup:simple syrup mixture with simple syrup, NF.

INSTRUCTIONS: Crush the tablets and triturate to a fine powder. Make a mixture of equal parts of syrup and methylcellulose. Add a small amount of this vehicle and levigate to a uniform paste. Add vehicle in geometric proportions almost to volume, mix thoroughly, and transfer to a graduate. Rinse the mortar with vehicle, add to the graduate, and qs to 100 mL.

NOTES

GENERIC NAME	**Alprazolam**
DOSAGE FORM	oral suspension
MADE FROM	tablets
CONCENTRATION	1 mg/mL
STABILITY	60 days
STABILITY REFERENCE	Allen LV Jr, et al. Am J Health Syst Pharm 1998; 55:1915-20
STORE	refrigerate (preferable) or at room temperature
LABEL	

INGREDIENT	STRENGTH	QUANTITY
Alprazolam tablets	2 mg	60
Ora-Plus:Ora-Sweet or Ora-Plus:Ora-Sweet SF	1:1 mixture	qs 120 mL

NOTE: In this study, the formulation was stored in amber clear plastic (polyethylene terephthalate) prescription ovals. Commercially available as an oral solution, 1 mg/mL and 0.5 mg/5 mL.

INSTRUCTIONS: Crush the tablets and triturate to a fine powder. Add approximately 40 mL of vehicle and levigate to a uniform paste. Add vehicle in geometric proportions almost to volume, mix thoroughly, and transfer to a graduate. Rinse the mortar with vehicle, add to the graduate, and qs to 120 mL.

NOTES

GENERIC NAME	**Alprazolam**
DOSAGE FORM	oral suspension
MADE FROM	tablets
CONCENTRATION	1 mg/mL
STABILITY	60 days
STABILITY REFERENCE	Allen LV Jr, et al. Am J Health Syst Pharm 1998; 55:1915-20
STORE	refrigerate (preferable) or at room temperature
LABEL	shake well before use, refrigerate

INGREDIENT	STRENGTH	QUANTITY
Alprazolam tablets	2 mg	60
Cherry syrup (cherry syrup concentrate diluted 1:4 with simple syrup, NF)		qs 120 mL

NOTE: In this study, the formulation was stored in amber clear plastic (polyethylene terephthalate) prescription ovals. Commercially available as an oral solution, 1 mg/mL and 0.5 mg/5 mL.

INSTRUCTIONS: Crush the tablets and triturate to a fine powder. Add approximately 40 mL of vehicle and levigate to a uniform paste. Add vehicle in geometric proportions almost to volume, mix thoroughly, and transfer to a graduate. Rinse the mortar with vehicle, add to the graduate, and qs to 120 mL.

NOTES

GENERIC NAME	**Amiloride**
DOSAGE FORM	oral suspension
MADE FROM	tablets
CONCENTRATION	1 mg/mL
STABILITY	21 days
STABILITY REFERENCE	Fawcett JP, et al. Aust J Hosp Pharm 1995;25: 19-23
STORE	refrigerate
LABEL	shake well before use, refrigerate

INGREDIENT	STRENGTH	QUANTITY
Amiloride hydrochloride tablets	5 mg	10
Glycerin BP (alternatively use glycerin, USP)		20 mL
Sterile water		qs 50 mL

NOTE: In this study, the formulation was stored in amber plastic containers.

INSTRUCTIONS: Crush tablets in a mortar and reduce to a fine powder. Add small portions of glycerin BP and mix to a uniform paste. Add approximately 20 mL of sterile water while mixing to almost volume. Transfer to a graduate and qs to volume with sterile water.

NOTES

GENERIC NAME	**Amiloride**
DOSAGE FORM	oral suspension
MADE FROM	powder
CONCENTRATION	1 mg/mL
STABILITY	30 days
STABILITY REFERENCE	Fawcett JP, et al. Aust J Hosp Pharm 1995;25: 19-23
STORE	room temperature
LABEL	shake well before use

INGREDIENT	STRENGTH	QUANTITY
Amiloride hydrochloride powder		50 mg
Glycerin BP (alternatively use glycerin, USP)		20 mL
Sterile water		qs 50 mL

NOTE: In this study, the formulation was stored in amber plastic containers.

INSTRUCTIONS: Add small portions of glycerin BP to amiloride hydrochloride powder and mix to a uniform paste in a mortar. Add approximately 20 mL of sterile water while mixing to almost volume. Transfer to a graduate and qs to volume with sterile water.

NOTES

GENERIC NAME	**Amiloride**
DOSAGE FORM	oral suspension (with preservatives)
MADE FROM	tablets
CONCENTRATION	1 mg/mL
STABILITY	90 days
STABILITY REFERENCE	Fawcett JP, et al. Aust J Hosp Pharm 1995;25: 19-23
STORE	refrigerate
LABEL	shake well before use, refrigerate

INGREDIENT	STRENGTH	QUANTITY
Amiloride hydrochloride tablets	5 mg	10
Glycerin BP (alternatively use glycerin, USP)		20 mL
[a]Parabens	0.1 %	
Sterile water		qs 50 mL

[a]Methyl hydroxybenzoate 4 g, propyl hydroxybenzoate 1 g, propylene glycol qs 100 mL. Mix 2 mL of this solution to 100 mL of formulation to give parabens 0.1%.

NOTE:	In this study, the formulation was stored in amber plastic containers.
INSTRUCTIONS:	Crush tablets in a mortar and reduce to a fine powder. Add small portions of glycerin BP and mix to a uniform paste. Add the parabens solution and mix well. Add approximately 20 mL of sterile water while mixing almost to volume. Transfer to a graduate and qs to volume with sterile water.

NOTES

GENERIC NAME	**Amiloride**
DOSAGE FORM	oral suspension (with preservatives)
MADE FROM	powder
CONCENTRATION	1 mg/mL
STABILITY	90 days
STABILITY REFERENCE	Fawcett JP, et al. Aust J Hosp Pharm 1995;25: 19-23
STORE	room temperature
LABEL	shake well before use

INGREDIENT	STRENGTH	QUANTITY
Amiloride hydrochloride powder		50 mg
Glycerin, BP (alternatively use glycerin, USP)		20 mL
[a]Parabens	0.1%	
Sterile water		qs 50 mL

[a]Methyl hydroxybenzoate 4 g, propyl hydroxybenzoate 1 g, propylene glycol qs 100 mL. Mix 2 mL of this solution to 100 mL of formulation to give parabens 0.1%.

NOTE: In this study, the formulation was stored in amber plastic containers.

INSTRUCTIONS: Add small portions of glycerin BP to amiloride hydrochloride powder and mix to a uniform paste in a mortar. Add the parabens solution and mix well. Add approximately 20 mL of sterile water while mixing almost to volume. Transfer to a graduate and qs to volume with sterile water.

NOTES

GENERIC NAME	**Aminophylline**
DOSAGE FORM	injection
MADE FROM	injection
CONCENTRATION	5 mg/mL
STABILITY	91 days
STABILITY REFERENCE	Nahata MC, et al. Am J Hosp Pharm 1992;49: 2962-3, Swerling R. Am J Hosp Pharm 1981;38: 1359-60
STORE	refrigerate
LABEL	refrigerate

INGREDIENT	STRENGTH	QUANTITY
Aminophylline injection	250 mg/10 mL	2 mL
Bacteriostatic water for injection, USP		8 mL

NOTE: In this study, the formulation was stored in plastic syringes.

INSTRUCTIONS: Add aminophylline injection to a 10-mL empty sterile vial and add bacteriostatic water for injection in a laminar flow hood.

NOTES

GENERIC NAME	**5-Aminosalicylic Acid**
DOSAGE FORM	enema (suspension)
MADE FROM	5-aminosalicylic acid powder (95%)
CONCENTRATION	100 mg/2.5 mL
STABILITY	90 days
STABILITY REFERENCE	Montgomery HA, et al. Am J Hosp Pharm 1986; 43:118-20
STORE	room temperature
LABEL	shake well before use, for rectal use only

INGREDIENT	STRENGTH	QUANTITY
5-Aminosalicylic acid	95%	168 g
Sodium phosphate dibasic (anhydrous)	1.6 g	
Sodium phosphate monobasic (anhydrous)	17.9 g	
Sodium chloride	36 g	
Sodium ascorbate	2 g	
Tragacanth	16 g	
Methylparabens	8 g	
Propylparabens	2 g	
Propylene glycol		100 mL
Distilled water		qs 4000 mL

NOTE: In this study, the formulation was stored in amber glass bottles.

INSTRUCTIONS: Add methylparaben and propylparaben to 100 mL of propylene glycol. Stir until dissolved. Pour approximately 3 L of water into a 4000-mL capacity blender. Add all other ingredients, including parabens solution. Blend on low speed for 1–2 minutes. Measure, add water, and qs to 4000 mL. Pour into gallon bottle and label.

NOTES

GENERIC NAME	**Amiodarone**
DOSAGE FORM	oral suspension
MADE FROM	tablets
CONCENTRATION	5 mg/mL
STABILITY	91 days
STABILITY REFERENCE	Nahata MC, et al. J Pediatr Pharm Pract 1999;4: 186-9
STORE	refrigerate
LABEL	shake well before use, refrigerate

INGREDIENT	STRENGTH	QUANTITY
Amiodarone tablets	200 mg	5
Ora-Sweet or Ora-Sweet SF		100 mL
Ora-Plus		100 mL

NOTE:	In this study, the formulation was stored in plastic prescription bottles. Adjust the Ora-Plus:Ora-Sweet SF formulation to pH 6–7 with sodium bicarbonate solution.
INSTRUCTIONS:	Mix Ora-Sweet (or Ora-Sweet SF):Ora-Plus in 1:1 proportion to obtain sufficient amount of vehicle. Crush the tablets in a mortar and reduce to a fine powder. Add small amounts of the vehicle to the mortar and levigate to a uniform paste. Add geometric proportions of the vehicle almost to volume. Transfer to a graduate and qs to 200 mL with vehicle while mixing.

NOTES

GENERIC NAME	**Amiodarone**
DOSAGE FORM	oral suspension
MADE FROM	tablets
CONCENTRATION	5 mg/mL
STABILITY	91 days (4 °C); 42 days (25 °C)
STABILITY REFERENCE	Nahata MC. Ann Pharmacother 1997;31: 851-2
STORE	refrigerate
LABEL	shake well before use, refrigerate

INGREDIENT	STRENGTH	QUANTITY
Amiodarone hydrochloride tablets	200 mg	3
Methylcellulose	1%	
Simple syrup, NF (50:50, v/v)		qs 120 mL

NOTE: In this study, the formulation was stored in plastic prescription bottles.

INSTRUCTIONS: Crush the tablets in a mortar and triturate well. Add the methylcellulose/syrup mixture vehicle in small amounts and levigate to form a uniform paste. Add more vehicle in geometric proportions, mix well, and transfer to a graduate. Rinse the mortar with the vehicle and qs to 120 mL.

NOTES

GENERIC NAME	**Amitriptyline**
DOSAGE FORM	oral liquid
MADE FROM	powder
CONCENTRATION	1 mg/mL
STABILITY	14 days
STABILITY REFERENCE	Amitriptyline hydrochloride 1-mg/mL oral liquid and gel. Int J Pharmaceut Compd 1999;3:218
STORE	refrigerate, protect from light
LABEL	refrigerate, protect from light

INGREDIENT	STRENGTH	QUANTITY
Amitriptyline hydrochloride		100 mg
Glycerin, USP		2 mL
Flavor		qs
Simple syrup, NF		qs 100 mL

NOTE: Stability-indicating analytical studies not used. Based on *United States Pharmacopeia XXIII/National Formulary 18* (Rockville, MD: US Pharmacopeial Convention, 1995:3531-5) beyond-use date for water-containing formulations in the absence of stability information.

INSTRUCTIONS: Levigate amitriptyline hydrochloride and the flavor with glycerin in a mortar to form a uniform paste. Add simple syrup almost to volume, mix well, and transfer to a graduate. Rinse the mortar with syrup, add to graduate, and qs to 100 mL.

NOTES

GENERIC NAME	**Amitriptyline**
DOSAGE FORM	oral suspension
MADE FROM	tablets
CONCENTRATION	20 mg/mL
STABILITY	42 days when refrigerated, 28 days at room temperature
STABILITY REFERENCE	Nahata MC, et al. Presented at: American Society of Health-System Pharmacists Midyear Clinical Meeting, December 2004 (poster)
STORE	refrigerate
LABEL	refrigerate, shake well before use

INGREDIENT	STRENGTH	QUANTITY
Amitriptyline tablets	100 mg	24
Simple syrup NF:	1:5	qs 120 mL
1% methylcellulose suspension		

NOTE: This formulation was stored in amber prescription bottles.

INSTRUCTIONS: Mix simple syrup and 1% methylcellulose suspension together thoroughly in a glass mortar pestle, in geometric proportions, to prepare the vehicle. Triturate the tablets into a fine powder and levigate with small proportion of the vehicle into a smooth suspension. Add vehicle in geometric proportions with constant mixing. Transfer to a graduate. Rinse the mortar and pestle with sufficient vehicle and transfer to graduate to make up the final volume.

NOTES

GENERIC NAME	**Amitriptyline**
DOSAGE FORM	oral suspension
MADE FROM	tablets
CONCENTRATION	20 mg/mL
STABILITY	91 days
STABILITY REFERENCE	Nahata MC, et al. Presented at: American Society of Health-System Pharmacists Midyear Clinical Meeting, December 2004 (poster)
STORE	refrigerate or room temperature
LABEL	refrigerate, shake well before use

INGREDIENT	STRENGTH	QUANTITY
Amitriptyline tablets	100 mg	24
Ora-Plus:Ora-Sweet	1:1	qs 120 mL

NOTE: This formulation was stored in amber prescription bottles.
INSTRUCTIONS: Mix Ora-Plus and Ora-Sweet together thoroughly in a glass mortar pestle, in geometric proportions, to prepare the vehicle. Triturate the tablets into a fine powder and levigate with small proportion of the vehicle into a smooth suspension. Add vehicle in geometric proportions, with constant mixing. Transfer to a graduate. Rinse the mortar and pestle with sufficient vehicle and transfer to graduate to make up the final volume.

NOTES

GENERIC NAME	**Amlodipine**
DOSAGE FORM	oral suspension
MADE FROM	tablets
CONCENTRATION	1 mg/mL
STABILITY	91 days (4 °C); 56 days (25 °C)
STABILITY REFERENCE	Nahata MC, et al. J Am Pharm Assoc 1999;39: 375-7
STORE	refrigerate
LABEL	shake well before use, refrigerate

INGREDIENT	STRENGTH	QUANTITY
Amlodipine tablets	5 mg	50
Methylcellulose	1%	125 mL
Simple syrup, NF		125 mL

NOTE: In this study, the formulation was stored in amber plastic prescription bottles.

INSTRUCTIONS: Crush the tablets in a mortar and triturate to a fine powder. Mix the syrup and methylcellulose thoroughly in a graduate. Add a small amount of the vehicle to the powder and mix to make a paste. Add the remaining vehicle in small quantities while mixing.

NOTES

Amlodipine

GENERIC NAME	**Amlodipine**
DOSAGE FORM	oral suspension
MADE FROM	tablets
CONCENTRATION	1 mg/mL
STABILITY	91 days (4 °C); 56 days (25 °C)
STABILITY REFERENCE	Nahata MC, et al. J Am Pharm Assoc 1999;39: 375-7
STORE	refrigerate
LABEL	shake well before use, refrigerate

INGREDIENT	STRENGTH	QUANTITY
Amlodipine tablets	5 mg	50
Ora-Sweet		125 mL
Ora-Plus		125 mL

NOTE: In this study, the formulation was stored in amber plastic prescription bottles.

INSTRUCTIONS: Crush the tablets in a mortar and triturate to a fine powder. Mix the Ora-Sweet and Ora-Plus together in a graduate. Add a small amount of the vehicle to the powder and mix to make a paste. Add the remaining vehicle in small quantities while mixing.

NOTES

GENERIC NAME	**Amphotericin B**
DOSAGE FORM	nasal solution
MADE FROM	injection
CONCENTRATION	0.5%
STABILITY	7 days
STABILITY REFERENCE	Pesko LJ. Am Druggist 1991;204:72
STORE	refrigerate, protect from light
LABEL	refrigerate, protect from light, for inhalation use only

INGREDIENT	STRENGTH	QUANTITY
Amphotericin B injection	50 mg	1 vial
Sterile water for irrigation		10 mL

NOTE: Stability-indicating analytical studies not used. Based on *United States Pharmacopeia National Formulary 20* (Rockville, MD: US Pharmacopeial Convention). Sterility testing not performed.

INSTRUCTIONS: Reconstitute the vial with sterile water for irrigation under a laminar air flow hood using aseptic technique. Mix until all the solid matter is dissolved completely, forming a clear yellow solution. Dispense in a nasal spray bottle or reusable atomizer delivering 0.3 mL/spray.

NOTES

GENERIC NAME	**Amphotericin B**
DOSAGE FORM	oral suspension
MADE FROM	powder
CONCENTRATION	100 mg/mL
STABILITY	93 days
STABILITY REFERENCE	Dentinger PJ, et al. Am J Health Syst Pharm 2001;58:1021-4
STORE	room temperature
LABEL	protect from light, shake well before use

INGREDIENT	STRENGTH	QUANTITY
Amphotericin B USP powder		30 g
Sterile water for irrigation		90 mL
Sodium phosphate dibasic USP (anhydrous)		4.77 g
Sodium phosphate monobasic USP		2.88 g
Sodium benzoate USP		0.3 g
Sodium metabisulfite USP		0.45 g
Citric acid USP		2.25 g
Carboxymethylcellulose 1% solution		37.5 mL
Paraben solution		3 mL
Cherry flavor		1.2 mL
Glycerin USP		45 mL
Sterile water for irrigation		qs 300 mL

NOTE: This formulation was stored in amber polyethylene terephthalate prescription bottles with child-resistant caps.

INSTRUCTIONS: Prepare the suspending vehicle by using the following steps. Dissolve sodium phosphate dibasic USP (anhydrous), sodium phosphate monobasic, sodium benzoate, sodium metabisulfite, and citric acid in approximately 90 mL of sterile water for irrigation in a 250-mL glass beaker, with constant mixing and applied heat. To this, add the carboxymethylcellulose 1% solution and mix until a uniform solution is formed. Prepare the paraben solution by dissolving 1 g of methylparaben and 0.2 g of propylparaben in 10 mL of propylene glycol. With constant mixing, add 3 mL of the paraben solution to the carboxymethylcellulose solution, allowing each drop to disperse before adding the next drop. Mix 1.2 mL of cherry flavor with 45 mL of glycerin and add to above solution, with constant stirring. This step completes the preparation of the suspending vehicle.

Add 30 g of amphotericin B powder to a porcelain mortar. Add the suspending vehicle in small proportions to wet the powder and levigate the powder into a smooth paste. Add more suspending vehicle to be able to make a smooth suspension and transfer to a 500-mL beaker calibrated to 300 mL. Use 150 mL of vehicle, rinse the mortar and pestle repeatedly and transfer to the beaker. Dilute the amphotericin B suspension with remaining suspending vehicle, followed by sterile water for irrigation to a final volume of 290 mL. Adjust the pH of the suspension to 5.3 with 200 mg/mL citric acid solution. Add enough sterile water for irrigation to bring up the final volume to 300 mL and mix well.

NOTES

GENERIC NAME	**Aprepitant**
DOSAGE FORM	oral suspension
MADE FROM	capsules
CONCENTRATION	20 mg/mL
STABILITY	90 days
STABILITY REFERENCE	Dupuis LL, et al. Support Care Cancer 2009;17:701-6
STORE	refrigerate
LABEL	shake well before use, refrigerate

INGREDIENT	STRENGTH	QUANTITY
Aprepitant capsules	125 mg	16
Ora-Blend		qs 100 mL

NOTE: In this study, the formulation was stored in amber polyethylene terephthalate or glass bottles.

INSTRUCTIONS: Empty the contents of the capsule into a mortar and triturate the contents to a fine powder, using the pestle. This may take 10-15 minutes. Add a small amount of Ora-Blend to the powder and levigate into a smooth paste. Add more Ora-Blend in geometric proportions, mixing well, and transfer to a graduate. Rinse the mortar repeatedly with Ora-Blend, add to the graduate, and qs to 100 mL.

NOTES

GENERIC NAME	**Atenolol**
DOSAGE FORM	oral suspension
MADE FROM	tablets
CONCENTRATION	2 mg/mL
STABILITY	90 days
STABILITY REFERENCE	Patel D, et al. Int J Pharmaceut Compd 1997;1: 437-9
STORE	refrigerate
LABEL	shake well before use, refrigerate

INGREDIENT	STRENGTH	QUANTITY
Atenolol tablets	50 mg	4
Ora-Sweet SF		qs 100 mL

NOTE: Stability-indicating analytical methods not used.

INSTRUCTIONS: Crush the tablets and triturate to a fine powder. Add a small amount of glycerin and levigate to a uniform paste. Add vehicle in geometric proportions almost to volume, mix thoroughly, and transfer to a graduate. Rinse the mortar with vehicle, add to the graduate, and qs to 100 mL.

NOTES

GENERIC NAME	**Atenolol**
DOSAGE FORM	oral suspension
MADE FROM	tablets
CONCENTRATION	2 mg/mL
STABILITY	14 days
STABILITY REFERENCE	Patel D, et al. Int J Pharmaceut Compd 1997;1: 437-9
STORE	room temperature
LABEL	shake well before use

INGREDIENT	STRENGTH	QUANTITY
Atenolol tablets	50 mg	4
Simple syrup, NF		qs 100 mL

NOTE: In this study, the formulation was stored in amber-colored prescription bottles.

INSTRUCTIONS: Crush the tablets and triturate to a fine powder. Add a small amount of glycerin and levigate to a uniform paste. Add vehicle in geometric proportions almost to volume, mix thoroughly, and transfer to a graduate. Rinse the mortar with vehicle, add to the graduate, and qs to 100 mL.

NOTES

GENERIC NAME	**Atropine sulfate**
DOSAGE FORM	injection
MADE FROM	powder
CONCENTRATION	1 mg/mL
STABILITY	72 hours
STABILITY REFERENCE	Dix J, et al. J Toxicol Clin Toxicol 2003;41:771-5
STORE	refrigerate or room temperature or 32-36 °C
LABEL	protect from light

INGREDIENT	STRENGTH	QUANTITY
Atropine sulfate USP lyophilized		5 g
0.9% Sodium chloride solution for injection		qs

NOTE: In this study, the formulation was stored in perfluflex polyvinyl sodium chloride bags covered with amber occlusive cover to protect from light.

INSTRUCTIONS: Using sterile technique (under a laminar flow hood if in a pharmacy), reconstitute 5 g of atropine sulfate with 10 mL of 0.9% sodium chloride solution for injection, agitate to dissolve. Through a 0.45-micrometer filter, inject this (10 mL) solution into 1000 mL of 0.9% sodium chloride solution for injection, resulting in an atropine sulfate 5 mg/mL stock solution. Protect from light by covering with an amber bag. Using sterile technique, withdraw 100 mL from a 500-mL 0.9% sodium chloride solution for injection bag and discard. Withdraw 100 mL of the atropine sulfate 5-mg/mL stock solution and add into the 400-mL of 0.9% sodium chloride for injection bag, resulting in an atropine sulfate 1 mg/mL solution. Protect from light by covering with an amber bag.

NOTES

GENERIC NAME	**Atropine sulfate**
DOSAGE FORM	oral solution
MADE FROM	tablets
CONCENTRATION	0.1 mg/mL
STABILITY	14 days
STABILITY REFERENCE	experience
STORE	refrigerate

INGREDIENT	STRENGTH	QUANTITY
Atropine sulfate tablets	0.6 mg	3
Purified water USP		18 mL

NOTE: No information about the type of storage container is provided in this study.

INSTRUCTIONS: Dissolve tablets in water.

NOTES

GENERIC NAME	# Azathioprine
DOSAGE FORM	oral suspension
MADE FROM	tablets
CONCENTRATION	50 mg/mL
STABILITY	60 days
STABILITY REFERENCE	Allen LV Jr, et al. Am J Health Syst Pharm 1996; 53:1944-9
STORE	refrigerate (preferable) or at room temperature
LABEL	shake well before use, refrigerate

INGREDIENT	STRENGTH	QUANTITY
Azathioprine tablets	50 mg	120
Ora-Sweet or Ora-Sweet SF		
Ora-Plus		aa qs 120 mL

NOTE: In this study, the formulation was stored in amber clear plastic (polyethylene terephthalate) prescription ovals.

INSTRUCTIONS: Mix Ora-Sweet (or Ora-Sweet SF):Ora-Plus in 1:1 proportion to obtain sufficient quantity of vehicle. Crush the tablets and triturate to a fine powder. Add approximately 40 mL of vehicle and levigate to a uniform paste. Add vehicle in geometric proportions almost to volume, mix thoroughly, and transfer to a graduate. Rinse the mortar with vehicle, add to the graduate, and qs to 120 mL.

NOTES

GENERIC NAME	**Azathioprine**
DOSAGE FORM	oral suspension
MADE FROM	tablets
CONCENTRATION	50 mg/mL
STABILITY	60 days
STABILITY REFERENCE	Allen LV Jr, et al. Am J Health Syst Pharm 1996; 53:1944-9
STORE	refrigerate (preferable) or at room temperature
LABEL	shake well before use, refrigerate

INGREDIENT	STRENGTH	QUANTITY
Azathioprine tablets	50 mg	120
Cherry syrup (cherry syrup concentrate diluted 1:4 with simple syrup, USP)		qs 120 mL

NOTE: In this study, the formulation was stored in amber clear plastic (polyethylene terephthalate) prescription ovals.

INSTRUCTIONS: Crush the tablets and triturate to a fine powder. Add approximately 40 mL of vehicle and levigate to a uniform paste. Add vehicle in geometric proportions almost to volume, mix thoroughly, and transfer to a graduate. Rinse the mortar with vehicle, add to the graduate, and qs to 120 mL.

NOTES

GENERIC NAME	**Azathioprine**
DOSAGE FORM	oral suspension
MADE FROM	tablets
CONCENTRATION	10 mg/mL
STABILITY	84 days (5 °C); 56 days (room temperature)
STABILITY REFERENCE	Dressman JB, et al. Am J Hosp Pharm 1983;40:616-8
STORE	refrigerate
LABEL	shake well before use, refrigerate

INGREDIENT	STRENGTH	QUANTITY
Azathioprine tablets	50 mg	6
Methylcellulose	1% solution	10 mL
Simple syrup, NF		qs ad 30 mL

NOTE: Stability-indicating analytical methods not used. In the study, the formulation contained Cologel 33 mL and wild cherry syrup:simple syrup, NF (1:2) qs 100 mL of 10 mg/mL of the formulation. Cologel, a commercially available vehicle consisting of methylcellulose 9% solution, is no longer available. In the above formulation, Cologel can be substituted with methylcellulose 1% solution and the wild cherry syrup:simple syrup mixture with simple syrup, NF.

INSTRUCTIONS: Crush the tablets and triturate to a fine powder. Make a mixture of syrup and methylcellulose in equal parts. Add a small amount of this vehicle and levigate to a uniform paste. Add simple syrup in geometric proportions almost to volume, mix thoroughly, and transfer to a graduate. Rinse the mortar with simple syrup, add to the graduate, and qs to 30 mL.

NOTES

GENERIC NAME	**Baclofen**
DOSAGE FORM	oral suspension
MADE FROM	tablets
CONCENTRATION	10 mg/mL
STABILITY	60 days
STABILITY REFERENCE	Allen LV Jr, et al. Am J Health Syst Pharm 1996;53:2179-84
STORE	refrigerate (preferable) or at room temperature
LABEL	shake well before use, refrigerate

INGREDIENT	STRENGTH	QUANTITY
Baclofen tablets	10 mg	120
Ora-Sweet:Ora-Plus	1:1 mixture	qs 120 mL

NOTE: In this study, the formulation was stored in amber clear plastic (polyethylene terephthalate) prescription ovals.

INSTRUCTIONS: Mix cherry syrup concentrate with simple syrup in 1:4 proportion to obtain sufficient amount of the cherry syrup vehicle. Crush the tablets and triturate to a fine powder. Add approximately 40 mL of vehicle and levigate to a uniform paste. Add vehicle in geometric proportions almost to volume, mix thoroughly, and transfer to a graduate. Rinse the mortar with vehicle, add to the graduate, and qs to 120 mL.

NOTES

GENERIC NAME	**Baclofen**
DOSAGE FORM	oral suspension
MADE FROM	tablets
CONCENTRATION	10 mg/mL
STABILITY	60 days
STABILITY REFERENCE	Allen LV Jr, et al. Am J Health Syst Pharm 1996; 53:2179-84
STORE	refrigerate (preferable) or at room temperature
LABEL	shake well before use, refrigerate

INGREDIENT	STRENGTH	QUANTITY
Baclofen tablets	10 mg	120
Cherry syrup (cherry syrup concentrate diluted 1:4 with simple syrup, NF)		qs 120 mL

NOTE: In this study, the formulation was stored in amber clear plastic (polyethylene terephthalate) prescription ovals.

INSTRUCTIONS: Crush the tablets and triturate to a fine powder. Add approximately 40 mL of vehicle and levigate to a uniform paste. Add vehicle in geometric proportions almost to volume, mix thoroughly, and transfer to a graduate. Rinse the mortar with vehicle, add to the graduate, and qs to 120 mL.

NOTES

GENERIC NAME	**Baclofen**
DOSAGE FORM	oral suspension
MADE FROM	tablets
CONCENTRATION	5 mg/mL
STABILITY	35 days
STABILITY REFERENCE	Johnson CE, et al. Am J Hosp Pharm 1993;50: 2353-5
STORE	refrigerate
LABEL	shake well before use, refrigerate

INGREDIENT	STRENGTH	QUANTITY
Baclofen tablets	20 mg	15
Glycerin, USP		sufficient to wet the powder
Simple syrup, NF		qs 60 mL

NOTE: In this study, the formulation was stored in amber glass bottles.

INSTRUCTIONS: Crush tablets in glass mortar and triturate to a fine powder. Add sufficient glycerin, USP, to wet the powder, and levigate well to form a uniform paste. Add vehicle in geometric proportions and transfer to a graduate. Rinse the mortar with the vehicle, add to graduate, and qs to 60 mL.

NOTES

GENERIC NAME	**Bethanechol**
DOSAGE FORM	oral suspension
MADE FROM	tablets
CONCENTRATION	5 mg/mL
STABILITY	60 days
STABILITY REFERENCE	Allen LV, et al. Am J Health Syst Pharm 1998; 55:1804-9
STORE	refrigerate (preferable) or at room temperature
LABEL	shake well before use, refrigerate

INGREDIENT	STRENGTH	QUANTITY
Bethanechol tablets	50 mg	12
Ora-Plus:Ora-Sweet or Ora-Plus:Ora-Sweet SF	1:1 mixture	qs 120 mL

NOTE: In this study, the formulation was stored in amber clear plastic (polyethylene terephthalate) prescription ovals.

INSTRUCTIONS: Crush the tablets and triturate to a fine powder. Add approximately 20 mL of vehicle and levigate to a uniform paste. Add vehicle in geometric proportions almost to volume, mix thoroughly, and transfer to a graduate. Rinse the mortar with vehicle, add to the graduate, and qs to 120 mL.

NOTES

GENERIC NAME	**Bethanechol**
DOSAGE FORM	oral suspension
MADE FROM	tablets
CONCENTRATION	5 mg/mL
STABILITY	60 days
STABILITY REFERENCE	Allen LV, et al. Am J Health Syst Pharm 1998; 55:1804-9
STORE	refrigerate (preferable) or at room temperature
LABEL	shake well before use, refrigerate

INGREDIENT	STRENGTH	QUANTITY
Bethanechol chloride tablets	50 mg	12
Cherry syrup (cherry syrup concentrate diluted 1:4 with simple syrup, NF)		qs 120 mL

NOTE: In this study, the formulation was stored in amber clear plastic (polyethylene terephthalate) prescription ovals.

INSTRUCTIONS: Crush the tablets and triturate to a fine powder. Add approximately 20 mL of vehicle and levigate to a uniform paste. Add vehicle in geometric proportions almost to volume, mix thoroughly, and transfer to a graduate. Rinse the mortar with vehicle, add to the graduate, and qs to 120 mL.

NOTES

GENERIC NAME	**Bethanechol**
DOSAGE FORM	oral solution
MADE FROM	tablets
CONCENTRATION	1 mg/mL
STABILITY	30 days
STABILITY REFERENCE	Schlatter JL, et al. Ann Pharmacother 1997;31: 294-6
STORE	refrigerate
LABEL	refrigerate

INGREDIENT	STRENGTH	QUANTITY
Bethanechol chloride tablets	25 mg	4
Sterile water for irrigation		qs 100 mL

NOTE: Excipients may play a role in degrading the drug. In this study, the formulation was stored in amber glass bottles. Stability-indicating analytical methods not used.

INSTRUCTIONS: Place the tablets in a glass mortar and triturate to a fine powder. Transfer the entire contents to a 100-mL graduated cylinder. Add sterile water for irrigation and qs to 100 mL. Dissolve the drug by sonicating for 15 minutes. Filter the solution through a 0.22-μm filter to remove insoluble excipients.

NOTES

GENERIC NAME	**BPND Mouthwash**
DOSAGE FORM	oral liquid
MADE FROM	injection
STABILITY	6 months
STABILITY REFERENCE	experience

INGREDIENT	STRENGTH	QUANTITY
Bacitracin	50 000-unit vial	1
Polymyxin	500 000-unit vial	1
Neomycin	250 mg/mL	2.5 mL
Alcohol	95%	31.25 mL
Propylparabens		750 mg
Methylparabens		7.5 g
Diphenhydramine elixir		1875 mL
Purified water, USP		qs ad 3750 mL

INSTRUCTIONS: Dissolve parabens in alcohol and add to diphenhydramine elixir. Dilute the antibiotics and add to the diphenhydramine elixir, then qs with water in a graduate.

NOTES

GENERIC NAME	**Busulfan**
DOSAGE FORM	oral suspension
MADE FROM	tablets
CONCENTRATION	2 mg/mL
STABILITY	30 days
STABILITY REFERENCE	Allen LV. US Pharmacist 1990;15:94-5
STORE	refrigerate
LABEL	shake well before use, refrigerate

INGREDIENT	STRENGTH	QUANTITY
Busulfan tablets	2 mg	100
Simple syrup, NF		qs 100 mL

INSTRUCTIONS: Crush the tablets and triturate to a fine powder. Add approximately 20 mL of vehicle and levigate to a uniform paste. Add vehicle in geometric proportions almost to volume, mix thoroughly, and transfer to a graduate. Rinse the mortar with vehicle, add to the graduate, and qs to 100 mL.

NOTES

GENERIC NAME	**Caffeine**
DOSAGE FORM	injection
MADE FROM	powder
CONCENTRATION	10 mg/mL
STABILITY	24 hours
STABILITY REFERENCE	Nahata MC, et al. DICP 1989;23:466-7
STORE	refrigerate
LABEL	refrigerate

INGREDIENT	STRENGTH	QUANTITY
Caffeine powder		1 g
Bacteriostatic water for injection, USP		qs ad 100 mL

NOTE: Stability-indicating analytical methods not used. Commercially available as caffeine citrate injection 20 mg/mL.

INSTRUCTIONS: Dissolve the caffeine powder in the bacteriostatic water for injection in a clean glass graduate. Draw this solution into a plastic syringe, attach a sterile 0.22-µm filter, and filter into an empty sterile vial.

NOTES

GENERIC NAME	**Caffeine**
DOSAGE FORM	injection
MADE FROM	powder
CONCENTRATION	10 mg/mL (as caffeine base)
STABILITY	90 days
STABILITY REFERENCE	Eisenberg MG, et al. Am J Hosp Pharm 1984;41:2405-6
STORE	refrigerate
LABEL	refrigerate

INGREDIENT	STRENGTH	QUANTITY
Citrated caffeine powder		10 g
Sterile water for injection, USP		qs 500 mL

NOTE: Quarantine the product until sterility and pyrogen testing are completed. Stability-indicating analytical methods not used.
Commercially available as caffeine citrate injection 20 mg/mL.

INSTRUCTIONS: Dissolve the citrated caffeine powder in about 250 mL of sterile water for injection, USP. Transfer the solution into a 500-mL empty evacuated container (EEC). Add sterile water for injection and qs to 500 mL in the same EEC. Filter the solution through a 0.22-µm filter set into another 500-mL EEC, then transfer the solution into sterile, empty 10-mL vials. Autoclave the vials at 121 °C for 15 minutes and allow to cool.

NOTES

GENERIC NAME	**Caffeine**
DOSAGE FORM	oral solution
MADE FROM	powder
CONCENTRATION	10 mg/mL (as caffeine base)
STABILITY	90 days
STABILITY REFERENCE	Eisenberg MG, et al. Am J Hosp Pharm 1984;41:2405-6
STORE	refrigerate
LABEL	refrigerate

INGREDIENT	STRENGTH	QUANTITY
Citrated caffeine powder		10 g
Sterile water for irrigation, USP		250 mL
Simple syrup NF:cherry syrup	2:1	qs 500 mL

NOTE: Stability-indicating analytical methods not used. Commercially available as an oral solution of caffeine citrate 20 mg/mL.

INSTRUCTIONS: Dissolve the citrated caffeine powder in 250 mL of sterile water for irrigation, USP. Add a mixture of simple syrup:cherry syrup (2:1) and qs to 500 mL.

NOTES

GENERIC NAME	**Caffeine**
DOSAGE FORM	oral solution
MADE FROM	powder
CONCENTRATION	5 mg/mL (as caffeine base)
STABILITY	90 days
STABILITY REFERENCE	Hopkin C, et al. Br J Pharm Pract 1990;4:133
STORE	room temperature

INGREDIENT	STRENGTH	QUANTITY
Citrated caffeine powder		0.100 g
Citric acid		0.100 g
Distilled water		qs 10 mL

NOTE:	Stability-indicating analytical methods not used. Commercially available as an oral solution of caffeine citrate 20 mg/mL.
INSTRUCTIONS:	Dissolve the caffeine citrate powder and citric acid in water and qs to 10 mL.

NOTES

GENERIC NAME	**Calcitriol**
DOSAGE FORM	oral liquid
MADE FROM	capsules
CONCENTRATION	0.02 mcg/mL
STABILITY	7 days
STABILITY REFERENCE	experience
STORE	refrigerate (preferred) or room temperature, protect from light
LABEL	refrigerate, protect from light

INGREDIENT	STRENGTH	QUANTITY
Rocaltrol capsule	0.25 mcg	0.36 mL
Corn oil, USP		25 mL

NOTE: Rocaltrol liquid-filled capsules: 0.25-mcg capsule contains 0.25 mcg per 0.17 mL and 0.5-mcg capsule contains 0.5 mcg per 0.17 mL. Wrap the amber glass bottle in foil and store in an amber bag.

INSTRUCTIONS: Puncture and withdraw the contents of a capsule with an 18-gauge needle and syringe. Repeat the process on the second and third capsules to make up a volume of 0.36 mL and transfer to an amber glass bottle. Add 25 mL of corn oil and mix well.

NOTES

GENERIC NAME	**Captopril**
DOSAGE FORM	oral solution
MADE FROM	tablets
CONCENTRATION	1 mg/mL
STABILITY	56 days (4 °C); 28 days (22 °C)
STABILITY REFERENCE	Nahata MC, et al. Am J Hosp Pharm 1994;51: 95-6, Nahata MC, et al. Am J Hosp Pharm 1994; 51:1707-8
STORE	refrigerate
LABEL	shake well before use, refrigerate

INGREDIENT	STRENGTH	QUANTITY
Captopril tablets	50 mg	2
Ascorbic acid tablet	500 mg	1
Distilled water		qs 100 mL

NOTE: In these studies, the formulation was stored in glass prescription bottles. A sulfur-like odor is not indicative of captopril degradation.

INSTRUCTIONS: Allow two tablets of captopril 50 mg to dissolve in 50 mL of water in a graduate. Add the ascorbic acid tablet and allow it to dissolve. Add distilled water and qs the mixture to 100 mL. Shake well to disperse. Do not filter.

NOTES

GENERIC NAME	**Captopril**
DOSAGE FORM	oral solution
MADE FROM	tablets
CONCENTRATION	1 mg/mL
STABILITY	56 days (4 °C); 14 days (22 °C)
STABILITY REFERENCE	Nahata MC, et al. Am J Hosp Pharm 1994;51: 95-6, Nahata MC, et al. Am J Hosp Pharm 1994; 51:1707-8
STORE	refrigerate
LABEL	shake well before use, refrigerate

INGREDIENT	STRENGTH	QUANTITY
Captopril tablets	50 mg	2
Sodium ascorbate injection	500 mg	1
Distilled water		qs 100 mL

NOTE: In these studies, the formulation was stored in glass prescription bottles. A sulfur-like odor is not indicative of captopril degradation.

INSTRUCTIONS: Allow two tablets of captopril 50 mg to dissolve in 50 mL of water in a graduate. Add the contents of a 500-mg ampul of sodium ascorbate and allow to mix well. Add distilled water and qs the mixture to 100 mL. Shake well to disperse. Do not filter.

NOTES

GENERIC NAME	**Carbamazepine**
DOSAGE FORM	oral suspension
MADE FROM	tablets
CONCENTRATION	40 mg/mL
STABILITY	90 days
STABILITY REFERENCE	Burckart GJ, et al. Am J Hosp Pharm 1981;38:1929-31
STORE	refrigerate (preferable) or at room temperature
LABEL	shake well before use, refrigerate

INGREDIENT	STRENGTH	QUANTITY
Carbamazepine tablets	200 mg	20
Simple syrup, NF		qs 100 mL

NOTE: Stability-indicating analytical methods not used. In this study, the formulation was stored in amber glass bottles. Commercially available as an oral suspension, 100 mg/5 mL.

INSTRUCTIONS: Crush the tablets using a mortar and pestle and reduce to a fine powder. Add small portions of the vehicle and mix into a uniform paste. Add the vehicle in geometric proportions almost to desired volume. Transfer to a graduate and qs to 100 mL with the vehicle.

NOTES

GENERIC NAME	**Carboxymethylcellulose Sodium**
DOSAGE FORM	oral suspension
MADE FROM	powder
CONCENTRATION	1.5%
STABILITY	6 months
STABILITY REFERENCE	experience
STORE	room temperature
LABEL	shake well before use

INGREDIENT	STRENGTH	QUANTITY
Carboxymethylcellulose powder	high viscosity	15 g
Alcohol, USP	95%	53 mL
Purified water, USP (cold)		qs ad 1000 mL

INSTRUCTIONS: Mix the ethanol and carboxymethylcellulose powder to make a slurry. Add this to 800 mL of cold water while stirring rapidly, then qs to 1 L with water. Allow to stand until clear.

NOTES

GENERIC NAME	**Carisoprodol**
DOSAGE FORM	oral suspension
MADE FROM	tablets
CONCENTRATION	350 mg/mL
STABILITY	14 days
STABILITY REFERENCE	experience
STORE	refrigerate, amber glass bottle
LABEL	shake well before use, refrigerate

INGREDIENT	STRENGTH	QUANTITY
Carisoprodol tablets (SOMA)	350 mg	60
Distilled water		10 mL
Cherry syrup, USP		qs 60 mL

NOTE: The formulation needs to be stored in amber glass bottles.

INSTRUCTIONS: Triturate tablets into a fine powder in a glass mortar. Add small quantities of distilled water in geometric proportions and levigate the powder into a smooth suspension. Add syrup in geometric proportions and levigate until a uniform mixture is formed. Transfer the suspension to a conical graduate. Rinse the mortar with sufficient syrup and transfer to the graduate. Repeat rinsing and add to graduate to qs to final volume. Pour into an amber glass bottle and shake vigorously.

NOTES

GENERIC NAME	**Carvedilol**
DOSAGE FORM	oral suspension
MADE FROM	tablets
CONCENTRATION	0.5 mg/mL
STABILITY	30 days
STABILITY REFERENCE	experience
STORE	refrigerate (preferred) or room temperature
LABEL	shake well before use, refrigerate

INGREDIENT	STRENGTH	QUANTITY
Carvedilol tablets	12.5 mg	4
Ora-Plus		30 mL
Ora-Sweet		qs 100 mL

INSTRUCTIONS: Triturate tablets into a fine powder in a glass mortar. Add small quantities of Ora-Plus in geometric proportions and levigate the powder into a smooth suspension. Transfer the suspension to a graduate. Rinse the mortar with sufficient Ora-Sweet and transfer to the graduate. Repeat rinsing and add Ora-Sweet to graduate to qs to final volume.

NOTES

GENERIC NAME	**Carvedilol**
DOSAGE FORM	oral suspension
MADE FROM	tablets
CONCENTRATION	0.1 mg/mL
STABILITY	84 days
STABILITY REFERENCE	data on file, GlaxoSmithKline, Philadelphia, PA, per Lexi-Comp
STORE	room temperature, amber glass bottles
LABEL	shake well before use, protect from light

INGREDIENT	STRENGTH	QUANTITY
Carvedilol tablets	3.25 mg	1
Distilled water		5 mL
Ora-Plus		10 mL
Ora-Sweet		15 mL

INSTRUCTIONS: Triturate the tablet into a fine powder in a glass mortar. Add small quantities of distilled water in geometric proportions and levigate the powder into a smooth paste. Add Ora-Plus in geometric proportions and levigate into a uniform suspension. Transfer the suspension to a graduate. Rinse the mortar with sufficient Ora-Sweet and transfer to the graduate. Repeat rinsing with Ora-Sweet and add to graduate to qs to 30 mL.

NOTES

GENERIC NAME	**Carvedilol**
DOSAGE FORM	oral suspension
MADE FROM	tablets
CONCENTRATION	1.67 mg/mL
STABILITY	84 days
STABILITY REFERENCE	data on file, GlaxoSmithKline, Philadelphia, PA, per Lexi-Comp
STORE	room temperature, amber glass bottles
LABEL	shake well before use, protect from light

INGREDIENT	STRENGTH	QUANTITY
Carvedilol tablets	25 mg	1
Distilled water		5 mL
Ora-Plus		10 mL
Ora-Sweet		15 mL

INSTRUCTIONS: Triturate the tablet into a fine powder in a glass mortar. Add small quantities of distilled water in geometric proportions and levigate the powder into a smooth paste. Add Ora-Plus in geometric proportions and levigate into a uniform suspension. Transfer the suspension to a graduate. Rinse the mortar with sufficient Ora-Sweet and transfer to the graduate. Repeat rinsing with Ora-Sweet and add to graduate to qs to 30 mL.

NOTES

GENERIC NAME	**Cefazolin**
DOSAGE FORM	ophthalmic drops
MADE FROM	injection
CONCENTRATION	33 mg/mL
STABILITY	4 days
STABILITY REFERENCE	Leibowitz HM. Philadelphia: WB Saunders, 1984: 353-86
STORE	refrigerate
LABEL	refrigerate, for ophthalmic use only

INGREDIENT	STRENGTH	QUANTITY
Artificial tears		15 mL
Cefazolin injection	500 mg	1 vial
NaCl 0.9% for injection		2 mL

INSTRUCTIONS: Reconstitute a 500-mg vial of cefazolin with 2 mL of NaCl 0.9% for injection. Remove 2 mL of artificial tears from the 15-mL bottle. Add 2.2 mL of the cefazolin solution to the artificial tears bottle.

NOTES

GENERIC NAME	**Cefazolin**
DOSAGE FORM	ophthalmic drops
MADE FROM	injection
CONCENTRATION	50 mg/mL
STABILITY	28 days
STABILITY REFERENCE	Bowe BE, et al. Am J Ophthalmol 1991;111: 686-9
STORE	refrigerate
LABEL	refrigerate, for ophthalmic use only

INGREDIENT	STRENGTH	QUANTITY
Cefazolin injection	500 mg	1 vial
Methylcellulose artificial tears		qs to reconstitute

NOTE: Sterility testing not performed. Stability-indicating analytical methods not used.

INSTRUCTIONS: Reconstitute the injection under laminar flow hood with the artificial tears, using aseptic technique, to achieve a concentration of 50 mg/mL. Transfer the solution to sterile ophthalmic dropper bottles. American Society of Health-System Pharmacists' guidelines (Am J Hosp Pharm 1993;50:1462-3) for compounding ophthalmic products should be considered while preparing this formulation.

NOTES

GENERIC NAME	**Cefazolin**
DOSAGE FORM	ophthalmic drops
MADE FROM	injection
CONCENTRATION	33 mg/mL
STABILITY	28 days
STABILITY REFERENCE	Charlton JF, et al. Am J Health Syst Pharm 1998; 55:463-6
STORE	refrigerate
LABEL	refrigerate, for ophthalmic use only

INGREDIENT	STRENGTH	QUANTITY
Cefazolin injection	500 mg	1 vial
Liquifilm Tears		15 mL

NOTE: Sterility testing not performed. Stability-indicating analytical methods not used.

INSTRUCTIONS: Remove 15 mL of the artificial tears aseptically and use it to reconstitute cefazolin. Remove the solution aseptically and transfer to the original artificial tears bottle. American Society of Health-System Pharmacists' guidelines (Am J Hosp Pharm 1993;50:1462-3) for compounding ophthalmic products should be considered while preparing this formulation.

NOTES

GENERIC NAME	**Cefazolin**
DOSAGE FORM	ophthalmic drops
MADE FROM	injection
CONCENTRATION	3.4 mg/mL
STABILITY	7 days
STABILITY REFERENCE	Ahmed I, et al. Am J Hosp Pharm 1987;44:2287-90
STORE	refrigerate
LABEL	refrigerate, for ophthalmic use only

INGREDIENT	STRENGTH	QUANTITY
Cefazolin injection	500 mg	1 vial (0.17 mL)
Liquifilm Tears or Liquifilm Forte or Isopto Tears or Tearisol		4.83 mL

NOTE: Sterility testing not performed.

INSTRUCTIONS: Reconstitute a cefazolin vial with sterile NaCl 0.9% solution to obtain a concentration of 100 mg/mL. Mix 0.17 mL of this stock solution with 4.83 mL of the artificial tears solution in the original artificial tears bottle. The entire procedure should be conducted aseptically under a laminar air flow hood. American Society of Health-System Pharmacists' guidelines (Am J Hosp Pharm 1993;50:1462-3) for compounding ophthalmic products should be considered while preparing this formulation.

NOTES

GENERIC NAME	**Cefuroxime**
DOSAGE FORM	ophthalmic drops
MADE FROM	injection
CONCENTRATION	50 mg/mL
STABILITY	24 hours (25 °C); 14 days (8–10 °C); 28 days (4 °C)
STABILITY REFERENCE	Hebron B, et al. Int J Pharm Pract 1993;2:163-7
STORE	refrigerate
LABEL	refrigerate, for ophthalmic use only

INGREDIENT	STRENGTH	QUANTITY
Cefuroxime injection	750 mg	1 vial
Sno Tears		15 mL

NOTE: Preservative testing for *Pseudomonas aeruginosa*, *Candida albicans*, and *Staphylococcus aureus* was performed.

INSTRUCTIONS: Remove 15 mL of the artificial tears aseptically and use it to reconstitute cefuroxime to achieve a concentration of 50 mg/mL. Transfer the solution aseptically to the original artificial tears bottle. American Society of Health-System Pharmacists' guidelines (Am J Hosp Pharm 1993;50:1462-3) for compounding ophthalmic products should be considered while preparing this formulation.

NOTES

GENERIC NAME	**Cefuroxime**
DOSAGE FORM	ophthalmic drops
MADE FROM	injection
CONCENTRATION	50 mg/mL
STABILITY	28 days
STABILITY REFERENCE	Hebron B, et al. Int J Pharm Pract 1993;2:163-7
STORE	refrigerate
LABEL	refrigerate, for ophthalmic use only

INGREDIENT	STRENGTH	QUANTITY
Cefuroxime injection	750 mg	1 vial
Hypromellose PF		15 mL

NOTE: The preparation may change color from pale to bright yellow. Preservative testing for *Pseudomonas aeruginosa*, *Candida albicans*, and *Staphylococcus aureus* was performed.

INSTRUCTIONS: Remove 15 mL of the artificial tears aseptically and use it to reconstitute cefuroxime to produce a concentration of 50 mg/mL. Transfer the solution aseptically to the original artificial tears bottle. American Society of Health-System Pharmacists' guidelines (Am J Hosp Pharm 1993;50:1462-3) for compounding ophthalmic products should be considered while preparing this formulation.

NOTES

GENERIC NAME	**Cefuroxime**
DOSAGE FORM	ophthalmic drops
MADE FROM	injection
CONCENTRATION	50 mg/mL
STABILITY	14 days
STABILITY REFERENCE	Hebron B, et al. Int J Pharm Pract 1993;2:163-7
STORE	refrigerate
LABEL	refrigerate, for ophthalmic use only

INGREDIENT	STRENGTH	QUANTITY
Cefuroxime injection	750 mg	1 vial
Sodium chloride PF		15 mL

NOTE: Preservative testing for *Pseudomonas aeruginosa*, *Candida albicans*, and *Staphylococcus aureus* was performed.

INSTRUCTIONS: Remove 15 mL of the artificial tears aseptically and use it to reconstitute cefuroxime to produce a concentration of 50 mg/mL. Transfer the solution aseptically to the original artificial tears bottle. American Society of Health-System Pharmacists' guidelines (Am J Hosp Pharm 1993;50:1462-3) for compounding ophthalmic products should be considered while preparing this formulation.

NOTES

GENERIC NAME	**Chlorambucil**
DOSAGE FORM	oral suspension
MADE FROM	tablets
CONCENTRATION	2 mg/mL
STABILITY	7 days
STABILITY REFERENCE	Dressman JB, et al. Am J Hosp Pharm 1983;40: 616-8
STORE	refrigerate
LABEL	shake well before use, refrigerate, protect from light

INGREDIENT	STRENGTH	QUANTITY
Chlorambucil tablets	2 mg	60
Methylcellulose	1% solution	30 mL
Simple syrup, NF		qs 60 mL

NOTE: Stability-indicating analytical methods not used. In the study, the formulation contained Cologel 33 mL and wild cherry syrup:simple syrup, NF (1:2) qs 100 mL of 2 mg/mL of the formulation. Cologel, a commercially available vehicle consisting of methylcellulose 9% solution, is no longer available. In this formulation, Cologel can be substituted with methylcellulose 1% solution and the wild cherry syrup:simple syrup mixture with simple syrup, NF.

INSTRUCTIONS: Crush the tablets and triturate to a fine powder. Make a mixture of equal parts of syrup and methylcellulose. Add a small amount of this vehicle and levigate to a uniform paste. Add vehicle in geometric proportions almost to volume, mix thoroughly, and transfer to a graduate. Rinse the mortar with vehicle, add to the graduate, and qs to 60 mL.

NOTES

GENERIC NAME	**Chloroquine**
DOSAGE FORM	oral suspension
MADE FROM	tablets
CONCENTRATION	15 mg/mL
STABILITY	60 days
STABILITY REFERENCE	Allen LV Jr, et al. Am J Health Syst Pharm 1998; 55:1915-20
STORE	refrigerate (preferable) or at room temperature
LABEL	shake well before use, refrigerate

INGREDIENT	STRENGTH	QUANTITY
Chloroquine tablets	500 mg	3
Ora-Plus:Ora-Sweet or Ora-Plus:Ora-Sweet SF	1:1 mixture	qs 100 mL

NOTE: In this study, the formulation was stored in amber clear plastic (polyethylene terephthalate) prescription ovals.

INSTRUCTIONS: Crush the tablets in a mortar and reduce to a fine powder. Add approximately 15 mL of the vehicle to the mortar and mix to a uniform paste. Add vehicle in geometric proportions almost to volume while mixing. Transfer to a graduate and qs to volume with vehicle.

NOTES

GENERIC NAME	**Chloroquine**
DOSAGE FORM	oral suspension
MADE FROM	tablets
CONCENTRATION	15 mg/mL
STABILITY	60 days
STABILITY REFERENCE	Allen LV Jr, et al. Am J Health Syst Pharm 1998; 55:1915-20
STORE	refrigerate (preferable) or at room temperature
LABEL	shake well before use, refrigerate

INGREDIENT	STRENGTH	QUANTITY
Chloroquine tablets	500 mg	3
Cherry syrup concentrate diluted 1:4 with simple syrup, NF		qs 100 mL

NOTE: In this study, the formulation was stored in amber clear plastic (polyethylene terephthalate) prescription ovals.

INSTRUCTIONS: Crush the tablets and triturate to a fine powder. Add approximately 15 mL of vehicle and levigate to a uniform paste. Add vehicle in geometric proportions almost to volume, mix thoroughly, and transfer to a graduate. Rinse the mortar with vehicle, add to the graduate, and qs to 100 mL.

NOTES

GENERIC NAME	**Chloroquine**
DOSAGE FORM	oral suspension
MADE FROM	tablets
CONCENTRATION	10 mg chloroquine base/mL
STABILITY	4 weeks
STABILITY REFERENCE	Deseda CC, et al. Pediatr Infect Dis J 1994;13: 827-8
STORE	refrigerate (preferable) or at room temperature
LABEL	shake well before use, refrigerate

INGREDIENT	STRENGTH	QUANTITY
Chloroquine tablets	500 mg (300-mg base)	2
Sterile water for irrigation		
Cherry syrup, USP		qs 60 mL

NOTE: In this study, the formulation was stored in glass amber bottles. Stability-indicating analytical methods not used.

INSTRUCTIONS: Crush two tablets to a fine powder in a mortar after removing the film coating. Levigate with a small amount of sterile water for irrigation into a uniform paste. Add sufficient amount of cherry syrup in geometric proportions and levigate to a uniform mixture. Transfer the contents of the mortar to a graduate. Rinse the mortar with cherry syrup, add to graduate, and qs to 60 mL.

NOTES

GENERIC NAME	**Chlorothiazide**
DOSAGE FORM	oral suspension
MADE FROM	tablets
CONCENTRATION	50 mg/mL
STABILITY	30 days
STABILITY REFERENCE	Woods DJ. www.pharminfotech.co.nz/emixt
STORE	refrigerate
LABEL	shake well before use, refrigerate

INGREDIENT	STRENGTH	QUANTITY
Chlorothiazide tablets	500 mg	10
[a]Carboxymethyl-cellulose sodium		2 g
[b]Parabens	0.1%	
Glycerin		10 mL
Citric acid monohydrate		0.500 g
Water		qs to 100 mL

[a]Alternatively, use a base of methylcellulose 1%.
[b]Methyl hydroxybenzoate 4 g, propyl hydroxybenzoate 1 g, propylene glycol qs 100 mL. Mix 2 mL of this solution to 100 mL of formulation to give parabens 0.1%.

NOTE: Stability-indicating analytical methods not used. Commercially available as an oral suspension, 250 mg/5 mL.

INSTRUCTIONS: In a glass mortar, levigate carboxymethylcellulose with sufficient amount (5–10 mL) of water to form a uniform paste. Add approximately 40 mL of water to the paste in geometric proportions with vigorous levigation (preferably use a blender). Transfer this to an appropriate container for heating. Heat the dispersion to about 60 °C with moderate stirring until the carboxymethylcellulose dissolves. Allow to cool and stand for 1–2 hours to form a clear gel. Crush the tablets and triturate to a fine powder in the glass mortar. Levigate the tablet powder with glycerin to form a uniform paste. Add the carboxymethylcellulose gel in geometric proportions and mix well. Dissolve citric acid in about 5 mL of water. Add the parabens solution and the citric acid solution in geometric proportions and mix well. Transfer to the graduate. Rinse the mortar with water, add to graduate with stirring, and qs to 100 mL.

NOTES

GENERIC NAME	**Cholesterol**
DOSAGE FORM	oral suspension
MADE FROM	liquid
CONCENTRATION	150 mg/mL
STABILITY	180 days refrigerated; 90 days at room temperature
STABILITY REFERENCE	experience
STORE	refrigerate or room temperature
LABEL	shake well before use, refrigerate, protect from light

INGREDIENT	STRENGTH	QUANTITY
Cholesterol		75 g
Cherry syrup		80 mL
Ora-Plus		265 mL

NOTE: In this study, the formulation was stored in amber glass bottles. Cholesterol used is of food grade (USP/NF CAS 310-516-8000), needs to be refrigerated, and has an approximate composition of 97.5% of cholesterol, 2% desmosterol, and 0.5% lathosterol.

INSTRUCTIONS: Combine Ora-Plus and cherry syrup in geometric proportions. Transfer this to a commercial mixer (with whisk attachment) and add cholesterol in geometric proportions while constantly mixing with whisk. Transfer contents to amber glass bottle.

NOTES

Cholestyramine/Petrolatum

GENERIC NAME	Cholestyramine/Petrolatum
DOSAGE FORM	topical ointment
MADE FROM	powder
CONCENTRATION	20%
STABILITY	180 days
STABILITY REFERENCE	experience; White CM, et al. Ann Pharmacother 1996;30:954-6
STORE	
LABEL	for external use only

INGREDIENT	STRENGTH	QUANTITY
Cholestyramine light powder (80% anhydrous)		25 g
Petrolatum ointment base		75 g

NOTE: Stability indicating analytical method not used. The concentration of anhydrous cholestyramine may vary among different generic powder brands, requiring recalculation of formula. This formulation is based on the use of PAR PHARMACEUTICAL brand of Questran Light, which contains 4 g of anhydrous cholestyramine in 5 g of powder per packet.

INSTRUCTIONS: Weigh out the powder and the ointment base. On an ointment slab, geometrically mix the powder with the ointment base and levigate thoroughly to form a smooth paste. Continue incorporating the ointment base in geometric proportions, followed with thorough levigation to obtain a smooth paste.

NOTES

GENERIC NAME	**Cimetidine Hydrochloride**
DOSAGE FORM	injection
MADE FROM	injection
CONCENTRATION	15 mg/mL
STABILITY	42 days
STABILITY REFERENCE	Nahata MC, et al. Am J Hosp Pharm 1993;50: 2559-61
STORE	refrigerate
LABEL	refrigerate

INGREDIENT	STRENGTH	QUANTITY
Cimetidine hydrochloride injection	150 mg/mL	1 mL
Sterile water for injection, USP		9 mL

INSTRUCTIONS: Mix aseptically in a syringe and store in an empty sterile glass vial.

NOTES

Cimetidine Hydrochloride

GENERIC NAME	
DOSAGE FORM	oral suspension
MADE FROM	tablets
CONCENTRATION	60 mg/mL
STABILITY	17 days
STABILITY REFERENCE	Tortorici MP. Am J Hosp Pharm 1979;36:22, Sparkman HE. Am J Hosp Pharm 1979;36:600
STORE	refrigerate
LABEL	shake well before use, refrigerate

INGREDIENT	STRENGTH	QUANTITY
Cimetidine hydrochloride tablets	300 mg	24
Glycerin, USP		10 mL
Simple syrup, NF		qs 120 mL

NOTE: Stability-indicating analytical methods not used. Commercially available as oral liquid, 300 mg/5 mL, containing 2.8% alcohol.

INSTRUCTIONS: Stand the tablets in about 5 mL of sterile water for approximately 3–5 minutes to dissolve the film coating. (per Tortotici). Crush the tablets and triturate to a fine powder. Add glycerin and levigate to a uniform paste. Add vehicle in geometric proportions almost to volume, mix thoroughly, and transfer to a graduate. Rinse the mortar with vehicle, add to the graduate, and qs to 120 mL.

NOTES

GENERIC NAME	**Ciprofloxacin**
DOSAGE FORM	oral suspension
MADE FROM	tablets
CONCENTRATION	50 mg/mL
STABILITY	91 days (4 °C); 70 days (25 °C)
STABILITY REFERENCE	Nahata MC, et al. J Appl Ther Res 2000;3:61-5
STORE	refrigerate (preferable) or room temperature
LABEL	shake well before use, refrigerate

INGREDIENT	STRENGTH	QUANTITY
Ciprofloxacin tablets	500 mg	20
Ora-Sweet:Ora-Plus	1:1	aa qs 200 mL

NOTE: In this study, the formulation was stored in plastic prescription bottles.
Commercially available as an oral suspension, 50 mg/mL and 100 mg/mL.

INSTRUCTIONS: Crush tablets in a mortar and reduce to a fine powder. Combine 100 mL each of Ora-Sweet and Ora-Plus, mix well, and add in small amounts to the ciprofloxacin powder. Mix well. Transfer to a graduate. Rinse mortar with small quantities of vehicle and transfer to graduate to qs to volume.

NOTES

Copyright © 2011 Harvey Whitney Books

GENERIC NAME	**Ciprofloxacin**
DOSAGE FORM	oral suspension
MADE FROM	tablets
CONCENTRATION	50 mg/mL
STABILITY	91 days (4 °C); 70 days (25 °C)
STABILITY REFERENCE	Nahata MC, et al. J Appl Ther Res 2000;3:61-5
STORE	refrigerate (preferable) or at room temperature
LABEL	shake well before use, refrigerate

INGREDIENT	STRENGTH	QUANTITY
Ciprofloxacin tablets	500 mg	20
Methylcellulose 1%:simple syrup, NF	1:1	qs 200 mL

NOTE: In this study, the formulation was stored in plastic prescription bottles. Commercially available as an oral suspension, 50 mg/mL and 100 mg/mL.

INSTRUCTIONS: Crush the tablets in a mortar and reduce to a fine powder. Mix equal quantities of methylcellulose 1% and simple syrup to obtain the vehicle. Add a small amount of the vehicle to the mortar and levigate to a uniform paste. Add geometric amounts of the vehicle while mixing. Transfer to a graduate. Rinse the mortar with vehicle, transfer to the graduate, and qs to 200 mL. Stir well.

NOTES

GENERIC NAME	**Ciprofloxacin**
DOSAGE FORM	oral suspension
MADE FROM	tablets
CONCENTRATION	50 mg/mL
STABILITY	56 days
STABILITY REFERENCE	Johnson CE, et al. Int J Pharmaceut Compd 1998; 2:314-7
STORE	refrigerate (preferable) or at room temperature
LABEL	shake well before use, refrigerate

INGREDIENT	STRENGTH	QUANTITY
Ciprofloxacin hydrochloride tablets	750 mg	4
Ora-Plus:simple syrup, NF (1:1)		qs 60 mL

NOTE: In this study, the formulation was stored in plastic amber prescription bottles. Commercially available as oral suspension, 50 mg/mL and 100 mg/mL.

INSTRUCTIONS: Crush the tablets in a mortar and triturate to a fine powder. Add approximately 15 mL of vehicle and levigate to a uniform paste. Add 15 mL of the vehicle in geometric proportions, mix thoroughly, and transfer to a graduate. Rinse the mortar with the remaining vehicle, add to the graduate, and qs to 60 mL.

NOTES

GENERIC NAME	**Cisapride**
DOSAGE FORM	oral suspension
MADE FROM	tablets
CONCENTRATION	1 mg/mL
STABILITY	91 days (4 °C); 28 days (25 °C)
STABILITY REFERENCE	Nahata MC, et al. Ann Pharmacother 1995;29: 125-6
STORE	refrigerate
LABEL	shake well before use, refrigerate

INGREDIENT	STRENGTH	QUANTITY
Cisapride tablets	10 mg	20
Methylcellulose	1%	qs 200 mL
Simple syrup, NF		100 mL

NOTE: Available commercially only under Limited Access Protocol at a concentration of 1 mg/mL.

INSTRUCTIONS: Crush the cisapride tablets in a mortar and triturate to a fine powder. Mix the syrup and methylcellulose together and add a small amount to the powder while mixing. Continue to mix and add the liquid mixture until uniform. Transfer to a graduate and qs to volume. Store in an amber plastic container.

NOTES

GENERIC NAME	**Cisapride**
DOSAGE FORM	oral suspension
MADE FROM	tablets
CONCENTRATION	1 mg/mL
STABILITY	60 days
STABILITY REFERENCE	Allen LV Jr, et al. Am J Health Syst Pharm 1998; 55:1915-20
STORE	refrigerate (preferable) or at room temperature
LABEL	shake well before use, refrigerate

INGREDIENT	STRENGTH	QUANTITY
Cisapride tablets	10 mg	12
Ora-Plus:Ora-Sweet or Ora-Plus:Ora-Sweet SF	1:1 mixture	qs 120 mL

NOTE: In this study, the formulation was stored in amber clear plastic (polyethylene terephthalate) prescription ovals. Available commercially only under Limited Access Protocol at a concentration of 1 mg/mL.

INSTRUCTIONS: Crush the tablets and triturate to a fine powder. Add approximately 20 mL of vehicle and levigate to a uniform paste. Add vehicle in geometric proportions almost to volume, mix thoroughly, and transfer to a graduate. Adjust the pH of the suspension to 7 with sodium bicarbonate. Rinse the mortar with vehicle, add to the graduate, and qs to 120 mL.

NOTES

GENERIC NAME	**Cisapride**
DOSAGE FORM	oral suspension
MADE FROM	tablets
CONCENTRATION	1 mg/mL
STABILITY	60 days
STABILITY REFERENCE	Allen LV Jr, et al. Am J Health Syst Pharm 1998; 55:1915-20
STORE	refrigerate (preferable) or at room temperature
LABEL	shake well before use, refrigerate

INGREDIENT	STRENGTH	QUANTITY
Cisapride tablets	10 mg	12
Cherry syrup (cherry syrup concentrate diluted 1:4 with simple syrup, NF)		qs 120 mL

NOTE: In this study, the formulation was stored in amber clear plastic (polyethylene terephthalate) prescription ovals. Available commercially only under Limited Access Protocol at a concentration of 1 mg/mL.

INSTRUCTIONS: Crush the tablets and triturate to a fine powder. Add approximately 20 mL of vehicle and levigate to a uniform paste. Add vehicle in geometric proportions almost to volume, mix thoroughly, and transfer to a graduate. Adjust the pH of the suspension to 7 with sodium bicarbonate. Rinse the mortar with vehicle, add to the graduate, and qs to 120 mL.

NOTES

GENERIC NAME	**Clindamycin**
DOSAGE FORM	injection
MADE FROM	150 mg/mL injection
CONCENTRATION	15 mg/mL
STABILITY	90 days
STABILITY REFERENCE	Nahata MC, et al. Am J Hosp Pharm 1993;50: 2559-61
STORE	refrigerate, store in an empty sterile vial
LABEL	refrigerate

INGREDIENT	STRENGTH	QUANTITY
Clindamycin injection	150 mg/mL	1 mL
Sterile water for injection, USP		9 mL

INSTRUCTIONS: Mix in a sterile syringe.

NOTES

GENERIC NAME	**Clonazepam**
DOSAGE FORM	oral suspension
MADE FROM	tablets
CONCENTRATION	0.1 mg/mL
STABILITY	60 days
STABILITY REFERENCE	Allen LV Jr, et al. Am J Health Syst Pharm 1996; 53:1944-9
STORE	refrigerate (preferable) or at room temperature
LABEL	shake well before use, refrigerate

INGREDIENT	STRENGTH	QUANTITY
Clonazepam tablets	2 mg	6
Ora-Plus:Ora-Sweet	1:1	
or Ora-Plus:Ora-Sweet SF	1:1	aa qs 120 mL

NOTE: In this study, the formulation was stored in amber clear plastic (polyethylene terephthalate) prescription ovals.

INSTRUCTIONS: Crush the tablets and triturate to a fine powder. Add approximately 10 mL of vehicle and levigate to a uniform paste. Add vehicle in geometric proportions almost to volume, mix thoroughly, and transfer to a graduate. Rinse the mortar with vehicle, add to the graduate, and qs to 120 mL.

NOTES

GENERIC NAME	# Clonazepam
DOSAGE FORM	oral suspension
MADE FROM	tablets
CONCENTRATION	0.1 mg/mL
STABILITY	60 days
STABILITY REFERENCE	Allen LV Jr, et al. Am J Health Syst Pharm 1996; 53:1944-9
STORE	refrigerate (preferable) or at room temperature
LABEL	shake well before use, refrigerate

INGREDIENT	STRENGTH	QUANTITY
Clonazepam tablets	2 mg	6
Cherry syrup (cherry syrup concentrate diluted 1:4 with simple syrup, NF)		qs 120 mL

NOTE: In this study, the formulation was stored in amber clear plastic (polyethylene terephthalate) prescription ovals.

INSTRUCTIONS: Crush the tablets and triturate to a fine powder. Add approximately 10 mL of vehicle and levigate to a uniform paste. Add vehicle in geometric proportions almost to volume, mix thoroughly, and transfer to a graduate. Rinse the mortar with vehicle, add to the graduate, and qs to 120 mL.

NOTES

Copyright © 2011 Harvey Whitney Books

GENERIC NAME	**Clonazepam**
DOSAGE FORM	oral suspension
MADE FROM	tablets
CONCENTRATION	0.1 mg/mL
STABILITY	60 days
STABILITY REFERENCE	Roy JJ, et al. Int J Pharmaceut Compd 1997;1: 440-1
STORE	refrigerate
LABEL	shake well before use, refrigerate

INGREDIENT	STRENGTH	QUANTITY
Clonazepam tablets	0.5 mg	20
Sterile water for irrigation		3 mL
Vehicle (see Instructions)		qs 100 mL

NOTE: In this study, the formulation was stored in amber PVC bottles.

INSTRUCTIONS: To prepare the vehicle, create a methylcellulose 1% solution by dissolving 2 g of sodium benzoate in about 200 mL of boiling water and adding methylcellulose 10 g 1500 cps, stirring for several minutes. Add ice-cold water quickly and qs to 1000 mL. Continue stirring the mixture for 10 minutes and then transfer it to a 1-L bottle. Store the bottle on its side under refrigeration at least 4 hours, which changes the product to a clear gel. Mix 700 mL of the above methylcellulose 1% gel with 300 mL of simple syrup, NF, containing methylparaben 1.1 mg/mL to obtain the vehicle. Mix well and store for at least 4 hours.

Crush the tablets and triturate to a fine powder. Add sterile water for irrigation and levigate to a uniform paste. Add vehicle in geometric proportions almost to volume, mix thoroughly, and transfer to a graduate. Rinse the mortar with vehicle, add to the graduate, and qs to 100 mL.

NOTES

GENERIC NAME	**Clonidine**
DOSAGE FORM	oral suspension
MADE FROM	tablets
CONCENTRATION	0.1 mg/mL
STABILITY	28 days
STABILITY REFERENCE	Levinson ML, et al. Am J Hosp Pharm 1992;49: 122-5
STORE	refrigerate
LABEL	shake well before use, refrigerate

INGREDIENT	STRENGTH	QUANTITY
Clonidine hydrochloride tablets	0.2 mg	30
Purified water, USP		2 mL
Simple syrup, NF		qs 60 mL

NOTE: In this study, the formulation was stored in amber glass bottles.

INSTRUCTIONS: Crush the tablets in a glass mortar and reduce to a fine powder. Slowly add 2 mL of purified water, USP, and triturate to a fine paste. Add 15 mL of vehicle to the paste, triturate well, and transfer to a 100-mL graduate. Rinse the mortar with another 15 mL of syrup and transfer to the graduate. Repeat rinsing with enough vehicle so as to qs the liquid in the graduate to 60 mL.

NOTES

GENERIC NAME	**Clopidrogel bisulfate**
DOSAGE FORM	oral suspension
MADE FROM	tablets
CONCENTRATION	5 mg/mL
STABILITY	60 days
STABILITY REFERENCE	Skillman KL, et al. Am J Health Syst Pharm 2010;67:559-61
STORE	refrigerate or room temperature
LABEL	shake well before use, refrigerate

INGREDIENT	STRENGTH	QUANTITY
Clopidrogel bisulfate tablets	75 mg	4
Ora-Plus		30 mL
Ora-Sweet		30 mL

NOTE: In this study, the formulation was stored in amber glass bottles.

INSTRUCTIONS: Triturate 4 tablets into a fine powder in a glass mortar. Mix equal quantities of Ora-Plus and Ora-Sweet in geometric proportions, with constant stirring, to produce 60 mL. Using 30 mL of this mixture, levigate the powder into a smooth suspension, adding the vehicle in geometric proportions. Transfer the suspension to a 2-oz child-resistant, amber, plastic container. Rinse the mortar with sufficient vehicle into the bottle to bring the final volume in the bottle to 60 mL.

NOTES

GENERIC NAME	**Clopidrogel bisulfate**
DOSAGE FORM	oral suspension
MADE FROM	tablets
CONCENTRATION	7.5 mg/mL
STABILITY	60 days
STABILITY REFERENCE	Skillman KL, et al. Am J Health Syst Pharm 2010;67:559-61
STORE	refrigerate or room temperature
LABEL	shake well before use, refrigerate

INGREDIENT	STRENGTH	QUANTITY
Clopidrogel bisulfate tablets	75 mg	6
Ora-Plus		30 mL
Ora-Sweet		30 mL

NOTE: In this study, the formulation was stored in amber glass bottles.

INSTRUCTIONS: Triturate 4 tablets into a fine powder in a glass mortar. Mix equal quantities of Ora-Plus and Ora-Sweet in geometric proportions, with constant stirring, to produce 60 mL. Using 30 mL of this mixture, levigate the powder into a smooth suspension, adding the vehicle in geometric proportions. Transfer the suspension to a 2-oz child-resistant, amber, plastic container. Rinse the mortar with sufficient vehicle into the bottle to bring the final volume in the bottle to 60 mL.

NOTES

Cocaine

GENERIC NAME	Cocaine
DOSAGE FORM	topical solution
MADE FROM	powder and injection
CONCENTRATION	cocaine 40 mg/mL, tetracaine 10 mg/mL, epinephrine 0.25 mg/mL
STABILITY	30 days
STABILITY REFERENCE	Cocaine and tetracaine hydrochlorides and epinephrine topical solution. *United States Pharmacopeia XXIII/National Formulary 18*. Supplement 9. November 1998:4535-6.
STORE	refrigerate, in sterile, light-resistant containers
LABEL	refrigerate, protect from light, for external use only, do not use if a precipitate is present

INGREDIENT	STRENGTH	QUANTITY
Cocaine hydrochloride		4.0 g
Tetracaine hydrochloride		1.0 g
Epinephrine injection (1:1000)		25 mL
Benzalkonium chloride		10 mg
Edetate disodium		6.4 mg
NaCl 0.9%		35 mL
Purified water		qs 100 mL

INSTRUCTIONS: Dissolve the cocaine and tetracaine hydrochlorides in about 25 mL of purified water and add the epinephrine injection (1:1000). Separately dissolve an accurately weighed quantity of edetate disodium in NaCl 0.9% and dilute quantitatively and stepwise, if necessary, with NaCl 0.9% to obtain 35 mL of a solution containing 6.4 mg of edetate disodium. Similarly and separately, dissolve an accurately weighed quantity of benzalkonium chloride in purified water (or use an accurately measured volume of benzalkonium chloride solution). Dilute quantitatively and stepwise, if necessary, with purified water to obtain 10 mL of a solution containing 10 mg of benzalkonium chloride. Combine the three solutions and add sufficient purified water to measure 100 mL. Mix to produce the topical solution.

NOTES

GENERIC NAME	**Codeine phosphate**
DOSAGE FORM	oral syrup
MADE FROM	powder
CONCENTRATION	3 mg/mL
STABILITY	90 days
STABILITY REFERENCE	Dentinger PJ, et al. Am J Health Syst Pharm 2007;64:2569-73
STORE	room temperature
LABEL	protect from light

INGREDIENT	STRENGTH	QUANTITY
Codeine phosphate, USP		600 mg
Sterile water for irrigation, USP		2.5 mL
Ora-Sweet		qs 200 mL

NOTE: In this study, the formulation was stored in amber polyethylene terephthalate bottles with child-resistant caps.

INSTRUCTIONS: Add 600 mg of codeine phosphate, USP powder into a glass mortar. Add the sterile water for irrigation and mix to dissolve the powder. Add Ora-Sweet to the glass mortar in geometric proportions, with stirring. Continue stirring for at least 10 minutes or until the solution is clear. Transfer to amber polyethylene terephthalate bottle. Rinse the mortar with sufficient Ora-Sweet and transfer to the bottle to make up the volume to 200 mL.

NOTES

GENERIC NAME	**Cortisone Acetate**
DOSAGE FORM	oral suspension
MADE FROM	powder
CONCENTRATION	5 mg/5 mL
STABILITY	7 days
STABILITY REFERENCE	Woods DJ. www.pharminfotech.co.nz/emixt
STORE	refrigerate
LABEL	shake well before use, refrigerate

INGREDIENT	STRENGTH	QUANTITY
Cortisone acetate		100 mg
Polysorbate 80		0.5 mL
Base (see instructions)		qs 100 mL

NOTE: Polysorbate 80 is used to wet the tablets. If not available, use a small amount of ethanol. Stability-indicating analytical methods not used.

INSTRUCTIONS: Formula for the base: sodium carboxymethylcellulose 1 g, syrup 10 mL, methyl hydroxybenzoate 0.150 g, citric acid monohydrate 0.600 g, lemon spirit 0.25 mL, water qs 100 mL.
Dissolve methyl hydroxybenzoate and citric acid in hot water. Add the syrup and lemon spirit and make up to 75 mL with water, then add the sodium carboxymethylcellulose and mix. Allow to hydrate for approximately 1 hour, then prepare up to volume. Triturate the cortisone powder in a mortar. Wet the powder with polysorbate 80 and levigate to a smooth paste. Add the base in geometric proportions, mix well, and transfer to a graduate. Rinse the mortar with the base, add to graduate, and qs to 100 mL.

NOTES

GENERIC NAME	**Cyclophosphamide**
DOSAGE FORM	elixir (oral)
MADE FROM	injection
CONCENTRATION	2 mg/mL
STABILITY	14 days
STABILITY REFERENCE	Brooke D, et al. Am J Hosp Pharm 1973;30:618-20
STORE	refrigerate, in amber glass bottles
LABEL	refrigerate

INGREDIENT	STRENGTH	QUANTITY
Cyclophosphamide injection		200 mg
Aromatic elixir, USP		qs 100 mL

INSTRUCTIONS: Withdraw the liquid injection from the vial and qs with the elixir in a graduate.

NOTES

GENERIC NAME	**Cyclophosphamide**
DOSAGE FORM	oral suspension
MADE FROM	injection
CONCENTRATION	10 mg/mL
STABILITY	56 days
STABILITY REFERENCE	Kennedy R, et al. Ann Pharmacother 2010;44: 295-301
STORE	refrigerate (prefereble) or room temperature
LABEL	shake well before use, refrigerate

INGREDIENT	STRENGTH	QUANTITY
Cyclophosphamide 2g injection USP	2 g	1 vial
0.9% Sodium chloride for injection		100 mL
Ora-Plus		100 mL

NOTE: In this study, the formulation was stored in 3-mL amber polypropylene oral dispensing syringes.

INSTRUCTIONS: Reconstitute a cyclophosphamide 2-g injection USP vial with 100 mL of 0.9% sodium chloride solution to achieve a solution of 20 mg/mL concentration. Mix this solution with equal quantities of Ora-Plus in geometric proportions with constant stirring. Transfer to an amber polypropylene bottle.

NOTES

GENERIC NAME	**Cyclophosphamide**
DOSAGE FORM	oral suspension
MADE FROM	injection
CONCENTRATION	10 mg/mL
STABILITY	56 days
STABILITY REFERENCE	Kennedy R, et al. Ann Pharmacother 2010;44: 295-301
STORE	refrigerate (prefereble) or room temperature
LABEL	shake well before use, refrigerate

INGREDIENT	STRENGTH	QUANTITY
Cyclophosphamide 2 g injection, USP	2 g	1 vial
0.9% Sodium chloride for injection		100 mL
Simple syrup, NF		100 mL

NOTE: In this study, the formulation was stored in 3 mL amber polypropylene oral dispensing syringes.

INSTRUCTIONS: Reconstitute a cyclophosphamide 2 g injection USP vial with 100 mL of 0.9% sodium chloride solution to achieve a solution of 20 mg/mL concentration. Mix this solution with equal quantities of simple syrup in geometric proportions with constant stirring. Transfer to an amber polypropylene bottle.

NOTES

GENERIC NAME	**Cyclosporine**
DOSAGE FORM	ophthalmic solution
MADE FROM	injection
CONCENTRATION	1%
STABILITY	28 days
STABILITY REFERENCE	Froyland K. Eur Hosp Pharm 1999;5:159-61
STORE	room temperature
LABEL	shake well before use

INGREDIENT	STRENGTH	QUANTITY
Cyclosporine injection (Sandimmune)	50 mg/mL	98 g
Peanut oil USP		qs 551 g

NOTE: In this study, the formulation was stored in glass containers with built-in silicon dropper devices.

INSTRUCTIONS: The eye drops should be aseptically prepared in a HEPA-filtered laminar air flow hood. Sterilize peanut oil at 150 °C for 4 hours. Filter the cyclosporine injection through a 1-µm filter into an Erlenmeyer flask containing the peanut oil. Place the flask on a magnetic stirrer and remove the ethanol by introducing into the flask medical grade nitrogen gas through a 0.22-µm filter at a rate of 7 L/min. After purging the solution with nitrogen for approximately 1 hour, a 1% w/w of ethanol concentration can be achieved. This can be determined by calculating the weight loss of the flask. The resulting solution can be then dispensed into glass containers.

NOTES

GENERIC NAME	**Cyclosporine**
DOSAGE FORM	paste
MADE FROM	cyclosporine oral solution (Sandimmune)
CONCENTRATION	9.6 mg/g
STABILITY	31 days
STABILITY REFERENCE	Ghnassia LT, et al. Am J Health Syst Pharm 1995;52:2204-7
STORE	refrigerate (preferable) or room temperature in aluminum-lined ointment tubes
LABEL	refrigerate

INGREDIENT	STRENGTH	QUANTITY
Cyclosporine oral solution (Sandimmune)	100 mg/mL	20.2 mL
Ora-Base		191.2 g

NOTE: In this study, the formulation was stored in aluminum-lined ointment tubes.

INSTRUCTIONS: Weigh Ora-Base and place on an ointment tile. Measure 20.2 mL of cyclosporine oral solution. Add the solution to an equal volume of Ora-Base and levigate the solution into the base. Repeat mixing the base into the mixture in geometric proportions until the 2 ingredients are completely combined. Place the paste into a catheter-tip syringe barrel after removing the plunger. Replace the plunger and push into the barrel to remove any air trapped in the syringe. Determine the tare of a 10-g ointment tube. Add about 6 cu cm of paste to the ointment tube and weigh. Add paste until the net weight of the tube's content is 7 g. Use a spatula to flatten the end of each tube; fold end-over 3 times and crimp the folded end.

NOTES

GENERIC NAME	**Dantrolene**
DOSAGE FORM	oral suspension
MADE FROM	capsules
CONCENTRATION	25 mg/5 mL
STABILITY	2 days
STABILITY REFERENCE	experience
STORE	refrigerate
LABEL	shake well before use, refrigerate

INGREDIENT	STRENGTH	QUANTITY
Dantrolene capsules	100 mg	5
Citric acid powder	150 mg	
Purified water, USP		10 mL
Simple syrup, NF		qs ad 100 mL

INSTRUCTIONS: Dissolve citric acid powder in water. Mix contents of capsules with small amount of syrup. Add citric acid solution and qs with syrup.

NOTES

GENERIC NAME	**Dantrolene**
DOSAGE FORM	oral suspension
MADE FROM	capsules
CONCENTRATION	5 mg/mL
STABILITY	30 days (at 5 ± 3 °C and 25 ± 2 °C)
STABILITY REFERENCE	Fawcett JP, et al. J Clin Pharm Ther 1994;19:349-53
STORE	refrigerate (preferable) or at room temperature
LABEL	shake well before use, refrigerate, protect from light

INGREDIENT	STRENGTH	QUANTITY
Dantrolene capsules	50 mg	10
Citric acid monohydrate	150 mg	
Purified water, USP		10 mL
Syrup BP (containing 0.15% w/v methyl hydroxybenzoate)		qs 100 mL

NOTE: In this study, the formulation was stored in the dark in amber polyethylene terephthalate bottles with polypropylene caps without inserts.

INSTRUCTIONS: Place the capsule contents in the mortar and triturate with citric acid solution in water to a uniform paste. Add syrup in geometric proportions with mixing to obtain a uniform suspension. Transfer the mixture to a graduate and qs with syrup to 100 mL.

NOTES

GENERIC NAME	**Dantrolene**
DOSAGE FORM	oral suspension
MADE FROM	capsules
CONCENTRATION	5 mg/mL
STABILITY	30 days (at 5 ± 3 °C and 25 ± 2 °C)
STABILITY REFERENCE	Fawcett JP, et al. J Clin Pharm Ther 1994;19:349-53
STORE	refrigerate (preferable) or at room temperature
LABEL	shake well before use, refrigerate

INGREDIENT	STRENGTH	QUANTITY
Dantrolene capsules	50 mg	10
Citric acid	0.150 g	
Distilled water		10 mL
Simple syrup, NF		qs 100 mL

NOTE: In this study, the formulation was stored in amber plastic prescription bottles.

INSTRUCTIONS: Crush the tablets and triturate to a fine powder. Dissolve citric acid in distilled water. Add the citric acid solution to the powder mix in the mortar and levigate into a smooth paste. Add syrup in geometric proportions, mix well, and transfer to a graduate. Rinse the mortar with additional syrup, transfer to the graduate, and qs to 100 mL.

NOTES

GENERIC NAME	**Dapsone**
DOSAGE FORM	oral suspension
MADE FROM	tablets
CONCENTRATION	2 mg/mL
STABILITY	91 days
STABILITY REFERENCE	Nahata MC, et al. Ann Pharmacother 2000;34: 848-50
STORE	refrigerate (preferable) or at room temperature
LABEL	shake well before use, refrigerate

INGREDIENT	STRENGTH	QUANTITY
Dapsone tablets	25 mg	16
Ora-Plus:Ora-Sweet or Ora-Plus:Ora-Sweet SF	1:1	qs 200 mL

NOTE: In this study, the formulation was stored in amber plastic prescription bottles.

INSTRUCTIONS: Crush the tablets in a mortar and reduce to a fine powder. Add a small amount of the vehicle and mix to a uniform paste. Add geometric proportions of the vehicle almost to volume and transfer to a graduate, then qs to volume while mixing.

NOTES

GENERIC NAME	**Desmopressin**
DOSAGE FORM	intranasal solution
MADE FROM	standard strength
CONCENTRATION	0.033 mg/mL
STABILITY	30 days
STABILITY REFERENCE	experience
STORE	refrigerate
LABEL	refrigerate, for inhalation only

INGREDIENT	STRENGTH	QUANTITY
Desmopressin acetate solution	0.1 mg/mL	2.5 mL
NaCl 0.9% injection, USP (nonbacteriostatic)		5 mL

INSTRUCTIONS: Withdraw 2.5 mL of desmopressin solution form the bottle using a sterile needle and syringe and an aseptic techniques and transfer to an appropriate sterile container suitable for intranasal use. Add 5 mL of 0.9% sodium chloride aseptically. Mix.

NOTES

Dexamethasone Sodium Phosphate

GENERIC NAME	Dexamethasone Sodium Phosphate
DOSAGE FORM	injection
MADE FROM	injection
CONCENTRATION	1 mg/mL
STABILITY	28 days
STABILITY REFERENCE	Lugo RA, et al. Ann Pharmacother 1994;28: 1018-9
STORE	refrigerate
LABEL	refrigerate

INGREDIENT	STRENGTH	QUANTITY
Dexamethasone sodium phosphate	4 mg/mL	1 mL
Bacteriostatic NaCl injection	0.9%	3 mL

NOTE: Use only to prepare neonatal doses.
INSTRUCTIONS: Using sterile technique in a laminar flow hood, transfer the ingredients to a sterile empty vial and label.

NOTES

GENERIC NAME	**Diazepam**
DOSAGE FORM	oral suspension
MADE FROM	tablets
CONCENTRATION	1 mg/mL
STABILITY	60 days
STABILITY REFERENCE	Strom JG Jr, et al. Am J Hosp Pharm 1986;43: 1489-91
STORE	refrigerate (preferable) or at room temperature
LABEL	shake well before use, refrigerate

INGREDIENT	STRENGTH	QUANTITY
Diazepam tablets	10 mg	10
Sucrose		55 g
Ethanol	95%	3.6 mL
Magnesium aluminum silicate		2.0 g
Sodium carboxymethylcellulose (medium viscosity)		1.0 g
Propylene glycol		5.0 mL
Raspberry flavor		qs
Red color		qs
Purified water		qs 100 mL

NOTE: In this study, the formulation was stored in amber glass bottles.
Commercially available as an oral solution, 1 mg/mL and 5 mg/mL.

INSTRUCTIONS: Sprinkle magnesium aluminum silicate on ~25 mL of purified hot water, allowing each portion to thoroughly wet without stirring. Allow to stand, with occasional stirring, for 24 hours. Stir until a uniform suspension is formed. In a glass mortar, levigate carboxymethylcellulose sodium with a sufficient amount (5 mL) of water to form a uniform paste. Add approximately 20 mL of water to the paste in geometric proportions, with vigorous levigation (preferably use a blender). Transfer to a suitable container for heating. Heat the dispersion to about 60 °C with moderate stirring until carboxymethylcellulose sodium dissolves. Allow to cool, then stand for 1–2 hours to form a clear gel. Mix the flavor and the color with ethanol. Crush the tablets and triturate to a fine powder in the glass mortar. Levigate the tablet powder with propylene glycol into a uniform paste. Dissolve sucrose in approximately 30 mL of water. Add the magnesium aluminum silicate magma and sucrose solution to the carboxymethylcellulose sodium gel in geometric proportions. Add the alcoholic solution and mix well. Transfer to a graduate, rinse the mortar with water, transfer to the graduate, and qs to 100 mL. Stir well.

NOTES

GENERIC NAME	**Diazoxide**
DOSAGE FORM	oral suspension
MADE FROM	capsules
CONCENTRATION	5 mg/mL
STABILITY	7 days
STABILITY REFERENCE	Woods DJ. www.pharminfotech.co.nz/emixt
STORE	refrigerate
LABEL	shake well before use, refrigerate, protect from light

INGREDIENT	STRENGTH	QUANTITY
Diazoxide capsules	50 mg	10
Sodium carboxymethylcellulose (alternatively, use methylcellulose)		0.400 g
[a]Parabens	0.1%	
Ethanol	95% or 90%	7 mL
Glycerin		40 mL
Water		qs 100 mL

[a]Methyl hydroxybenzoate 4 g, propyl hydroxybenzoate 1 g, propylene glycol qs 100 mL. Mix 2 mL of this solution to 100 mL of formulation to give parabens 0.1%.

NOTE: Stability-indicating analytical methods not used. Commercially available as an oral suspension, 50 mg/mL.

INSTRUCTIONS: Triturate the capsule contents with approximately 10 mL of glycerin. Hydrate the sodium carboxymethylcellulose in about 25 mL of water and add this to the crushed capsule paste when cooled. Mix thoroughly, add the other excipients, and qs to volume.

NOTES

GENERIC NAME	**Diltiazem**
DOSAGE FORM	oral suspension
MADE FROM	tablets
CONCENTRATION	12 mg/mL
STABILITY	60 days
STABILITY REFERENCE	Allen LV Jr, et al. Am J Health Syst Pharm 1996; 53:2179-84
STORE	refrigerate (preferable) or at room temperature
LABEL	shake well before use, refrigerate

INGREDIENT	STRENGTH	QUANTITY
Diltiazem hydrochloride tablets	90 mg	16
Ora-Plus:Ora-Sweet or Ora-Plus:Ora-Sweet SF	1:1 mixture	qs 120 mL

NOTE: In this study, the formulation was stored in amber clear plastic (polyethylene terephthalate) prescription ovals.

INSTRUCTIONS: Crush the tablets and triturate to a fine powder. Add approximately 10 mL of vehicle and levigate to a uniform paste. Add vehicle in geometric proportions almost to volume, mix thoroughly, and transfer to a graduate. Rinse the mortar with vehicle, add to the graduate, and qs to 120 mL.

NOTES

GENERIC NAME	**Diltiazem**
DOSAGE FORM	oral suspension
MADE FROM	tablets
CONCENTRATION	12 mg/mL
STABILITY	60 days
STABILITY REFERENCE	Allen LV Jr, et al. Am J Health Syst Pharm 1996; 53:2179-84
STORE	refrigerate (preferable) or at room temperature
LABEL	shake well before use, refrigerate

INGREDIENT	STRENGTH	QUANTITY
Diltiazem hydrochloride tablets	90 mg	16
Cherry syrup (cherry syrup concentrate diluted 1:4 with simple syrup, NF)		qs 120 mL

NOTE: In this study, the formulation was stored in amber clear plastic (polyethylene terephthalate) prescription ovals.

INSTRUCTIONS: Crush the tablets and triturate to a fine powder. Add approximately 10 mL of vehicle and levigate to a uniform paste. Add vehicle in geometric proportions almost to volume, mix thoroughly, and transfer to a graduate. Rinse the mortar with vehicle, add to the graduate, and qs to 120 mL.

NOTES

GENERIC NAME	**Diltiazem**
DOSAGE FORM	oral solution
MADE FROM	powder
CONCENTRATION	1 mg/mL
STABILITY	50 days
STABILITY REFERENCE	Suleiman MS, et al. J Clin Pharm Ther 1988; 13:417-22
STORE	room temperature

INGREDIENT	STRENGTH	QUANTITY
Diltiazem hydrochloride powder		100 mg
Dextrose monohydrate		5.55 g
Double distilled water		qs 100 mL

NOTE: Stability-indicating analytical methods not used.

INSTRUCTIONS: Mix the weighed quantity of diltiazem and dextrose in a glass mortar in geometric proportions. Measure 25 mL of water, add to the mixture, and solubilize the mixture. Transfer the solution to a 100-mL graduate and qs with water to 100 mL.

NOTES

GENERIC NAME	**Diltiazem**
DOSAGE FORM	oral solution
MADE FROM	powder
CONCENTRATION	1 mg/mL
STABILITY	50 days
STABILITY REFERENCE	Suleiman MS, et al. J Clin Pharm Ther 1988;13: 417-22
STORE	room temperature

INGREDIENT	STRENGTH	QUANTITY
Diltiazem hydrochloride powder		100 mg
Fructose		5.04 g
Double distilled water		qs 100 mL

NOTE: Stability-indicating analytical methods not used.
INSTRUCTIONS: Mix the weighed quantity of diltiazem and fructose in a glass mortar in geometric proportions. Measure 25 mL of water, add to the mixture, and solubilize the mixture. Transfer the solution to a 100-mL graduate and qs with water to 100 mL.

NOTES

GENERIC NAME	**Diltiazem**
DOSAGE FORM	oral solution
MADE FROM	powder
CONCENTRATION	1 mg/mL
STABILITY	50 days
STABILITY REFERENCE	Suleiman MS, et al. J Clin Pharm Ther 1988;13: 417-22
STORE	room temperature

INGREDIENT	STRENGTH	QUANTITY
Diltiazem hydrochloride powder		100 mg
Sucrose		9.58 g
Double distilled water		qs 100 mL

NOTE: Stability-indicating analytical methods not used.

INSTRUCTIONS: Mix the weighed quantity of diltiazem and sucrose in a glass mortar in geometric proportions. Measure 25 mL of water, add to the mixture, and solubilize the mixture. Transfer the solution to a 100-mL graduate and qs with water to 100 mL.

NOTES

GENERIC NAME	**Diphtheria/Tetanus Toxoids, Adsorbed**
DOSAGE FORM	skin test
MADE FROM	vaccine
CONCENTRATION	1:100
STABILITY	30 days
STABILITY REFERENCE	Franz ML, et al. J Pediatr 1976;88:975-7
STORE	refrigerate
LABEL	refrigerate

INGREDIENT	STRENGTH	QUANTITY
Diphtheria/tetanus pediatric vaccine		0.1 mL
Bacteriostatic water for injection, USP		9.9 mL

INSTRUCTIONS: Add the ingredients to an empty sterile 10-mL vial. Package in 0.2-mL amounts into tuberculin syringes for skin test use.

NOTES

GENERIC NAME	**Dipyridamole**
DOSAGE FORM	oral suspension
MADE FROM	tablets
CONCENTRATION	10 mg/mL
STABILITY	60 days
STABILITY REFERENCE	Allen LV Jr, et al. Am J Health Syst Pharm 1996; 53:2179-84
STORE	refrigerate (preferable) or at room temperature
LABEL	shake well before use, refrigerate

INGREDIENT	STRENGTH	QUANTITY
Dipyridamole tablets	50 mg	24
Ora-Plus:Ora-Sweet or Ora-Plus:Ora-Sweet SF	1:1 mixture	qs 120 mL

NOTE: In this study, the formulation was stored in amber clear plastic (polyethylene terephthalate) prescription ovals.

INSTRUCTIONS: Crush the tablets and triturate to a fine powder. Add approximately 20 mL of vehicle and levigate to a uniform paste. Add vehicle in geometric proportions almost to volume, mix thoroughly, and transfer to a graduate. Rinse the mortar with vehicle, add to the graduate, and qs to 120 mL.

NOTES

GENERIC NAME	**Dipyridamole**
DOSAGE FORM	oral suspension
MADE FROM	tablets
CONCENTRATION	10 mg/mL
STABILITY	60 days
STABILITY REFERENCE	Allen LV Jr, et al. Am J Health Syst Pharm 1996; 53:2179-84
STORE	refrigerate (preferable) or at room temperature
LABEL	shake well before use, refrigerate

INGREDIENT	STRENGTH	QUANTITY
Dipyridamole tablets	50 mg	24
Cherry syrup (cherry syrup concentrate diluted 1:4 with simple syrup, NF)		qs 120 mL

NOTE: In this study, the formulation was stored in amber clear plastic (polyethylene terephthalate) prescription ovals.

INSTRUCTIONS: Crush the tablets and triturate to a fine powder. Add approximately 20 mL of vehicle and levigate to a uniform paste. Add vehicle in geometric proportions almost to volume, mix thoroughly, and transfer to a graduate. Rinse the mortar with vehicle, add to the graduate, and qs to 120 mL.

NOTES

Copyright © 2011 Harvey Whitney Books

GENERIC NAME	**Disopyramide**
DOSAGE FORM	oral suspension
MADE FROM	capsules
CONCENTRATION	1 mg/mL
STABILITY	28 days
STABILITY REFERENCE	Mathur LK, et al. Am J Hosp Pharm 1982;39:309-10
STORE	refrigerate (preferable) or at room temperature
LABEL	shake well before use, refrigerate

INGREDIENT	STRENGTH	QUANTITY
Disopyramide phosphate capsule	100 mg	1
Simple syrup, NF		qs 100 mL

NOTE: In this study, the formulation was stored in type III amber glass prescription bottles. The formulation was compounded using cherry syrup, NF.

INSTRUCTIONS: Empty contents of the capsule in a mortar. Add syrup in small amounts and levigate to a smooth paste. Add syrup in geometric proportions and transfer to a graduate. Rinse the mortar with syrup, add to graduate, and qs to 100 mL.

NOTES

GENERIC NAME	**Disopyramide**
DOSAGE FORM	oral suspension
MADE FROM	capsules
CONCENTRATION	10 mg/mL
STABILITY	28 days
STABILITY REFERENCE	Mathur LK, et al. Am J Hosp Pharm 1982;39: 309-10
STORE	refrigerate (preferable) or at room temperature
LABEL	shake well before use, refrigerate

INGREDIENT	STRENGTH	QUANTITY
Disopyramide phosphate capsules	100 mg	10
Simple syrup, NF		qs 100 mL

NOTE: In this study, the formulation was stored in type III amber glass prescription bottles. The formulation was compounded using cherry syrup, NF.

INSTRUCTIONS: Empty contents of the capsules in a mortar. Add syrup in small amounts and levigate to a smooth paste. Add syrup in geometric proportions and transfer to a graduate. Rinse the mortar with syrup, add to graduate, and qs to 100 mL.

NOTES

GENERIC NAME	**Dolasetron Mesylate**
DOSAGE FORM	oral suspension
MADE FROM	tablets
CONCENTRATION	10 mg/mL
STABILITY	90 days
STABILITY REFERENCE	Johnson CE, et al. Am J Health Syst Pharm 2003; 60:2242-4
STORE	refrigerate (prefereable) or room temperature
LABEL	shake well before use, refrigerate

INGREDIENT	STRENGTH	QUANTITY
Dolasetron mesylate tablets	50 mg	12
Ora-Plus		30 mL
Simple syrup, NF		101 mL
Strawberry fountain syrup		19 mL

NOTE: In this study, the formulation was stored in amber child-resistant prescription bottles.

INSTRUCTIONS: Prepare strawberry syrup by mixing simple syrup, NF, and strawberry fountain syrup in geometric proportions with constant stirring. Triturate 12 tablets into a fine powder in a glass mortar. Mix equal quantities of Ora-Plus and strawberry syrup (initially prepared) in geometric proportions, with constant stirring, to produce 60 mL. Using 15 mL of this mixture, levigate the powder into a smooth suspension, adding the vehicle in geometric proportions. Transfer the suspension to a 2-oz child-resistant amber prescription bottle. Rinse the mortar with sufficient vehicle, transfer into the bottle to bring the final volume to 60 mL.

NOTES

Dolasetron Mesylate

GENERIC NAME	**Dolasetron Mesylate**
DOSAGE FORM	oral suspension
MADE FROM	tablets
CONCENTRATION	10 mg/mL
STABILITY	90 days
STABILITY REFERENCE	Johnson CE, et al. Am J Health Syst Pharm 2003;60:2242-4
STORE	refrigerate or room temperature
LABEL	shake well before use, refrigerate, protect from light

INGREDIENT	STRENGTH	QUANTITY
Dolasetron mesylate tablets	50 mg	12
Ora-Plus		30 mL
Ora-Sweet SF		30 mL

NOTE: In this study, the formulation was stored in amber child-resistant prescription bottles.

INSTRUCTIONS: Triturate 12 tablets into a fine powder in a glass mortar. Mix equal quantities of Ora-Plus and Ora-Sweet SF in geometric proportions with constant stirring to produce 60 mL. Using 15 mL of this mixture, levigate the powder into a smooth suspension, adding the vehicle in geometric proportions. Transfer the suspension to a 2-oz child-resistant amber prescription bottle. Rinse the mortar with sufficient vehicle into the bottle to bring the final volume in the bottle to 60 mL.

NOTES

GENERIC NAME	**Doxycycline**
DOSAGE FORM	oral suspension
MADE FROM	tablets
CONCENTRATION	5 mg/mL
STABILITY	14 days
STABILITY REFERENCE	Nahata MC, et al. Presented at: American Society of Health-System Pharmacists Midyear Clinical Meeting, December 2005.
STORE	refrigerate or room temperature
LABEL	refrigerate, protect from light, shake well before use

INGREDIENT	STRENGTH	QUANTITY
Doxycycline tablets	100 mg	6
Simple syrup NF: 1% methylcellulose suspension	1:10	qs 120 mL

NOTE: This formulation was stored in amber prescription bottles.

INSTRUCTIONS: Mix simple syrup and 1% methylcellulose suspension together thoroughly in a glass mortar pestle, in geometric proportions, to prepare the vehicle. Triturate the tablets into a fine powder and levigate with small proportion of the vehicle into a smooth suspension. Add vehicle in geometric proportions, with constant mixing. Transfer to a graduate. Rinse the mortar and pestle with sufficient vehicle and transfer to graduate to make up the final volume.

NOTES

GENERIC NAME	**Doxycycline**
DOSAGE FORM	oral suspension
MADE FROM	tablets
CONCENTRATION	5 mg/mL
STABILITY	14 days
STABILITY REFERENCE	Nahata MC, et al. Presented at: American Society of Health-System Pharmacists Midyear Clinical Meeting, December 2005.
STORE	refrigerate or room temperature
LABEL	refrigerate, protect from light, shake well before use

INGREDIENT	STRENGTH	QUANTITY
Doxycycline tablets	100 mg	6
Ora-Plus:Ora-Sweet	1:1	qs 120 mL

NOTE: This formulation was stored in amber prescription bottles.

INSTRUCTIONS: Mix Ora-Plus and Ora-Sweet together thoroughly in a glass mortar pestle, in geometric proportions, to prepare the vehicle. Triturate the tablets into a fine powder and levigate with small proportion of the vehicle into a smooth suspension. Add vehicle in geometric proportions, with constant mixing. Transfer to a graduate. Rinse the mortar and pestle with sufficient vehicle and transfer to graduate to make up the final volume.

NOTES

GENERIC NAME	**Edetate Calcium Disodium with Procaine Hydrochloride**
DOSAGE FORM	injection
MADE FROM	injection
CONCENTRATION	150 mg/mL and 0.5%
STABILITY	3 months
STABILITY REFERENCE	experience
STORE	for intramuscular use only

INGREDIENT	STRENGTH	QUANTITY
Edetate injection	200 mg/mL	5 mL
Procaine injection	2%	1.67 mL

NOTE: Used in treating high lead concentrations.
INSTRUCTIONS: Add edetate calcium disodium and procaine to an empty sterile vial.

NOTES

GENERIC NAME	**Enalapril**
DOSAGE FORM	oral suspension
MADE FROM	tablets
CONCENTRATION	1 mg/mL
STABILITY	91 days (4 °C); 56 days (25 °C)
STABILITY REFERENCE	Nahata MC, et al. Am J Health Syst Pharm 1998; 55:1155-7
STORE	refrigerate
LABEL	shake well before use, refrigerate

INGREDIENT	STRENGTH	QUANTITY
Enalapril tablets	10 mg	20
Ora-Plus:Ora-Sweet	1:1	aa qs 200 mL

NOTE: In this study, the formulation was stored in plastic prescription bottles.

INSTRUCTIONS: Mix equal amounts of Ora-Plus and Ora-Sweet in geometric proportions to prepare the vehicle. Crush the tablets in a mortar and reduce to a fine powder. Add a small amount of vehicle and levigate to a uniform paste. Add increasing amounts of vehicle in geometric proportions, mix well, and make the suspension pourable. Transfer the suspension to a graduate. Rinse the mortar with vehicle, transfer the rinsings to the graduate, and qs to 200 mL.

NOTES

GENERIC NAME	**Enalapril**
DOSAGE FORM	oral suspension
MADE FROM	tablets
CONCENTRATION	1 mg/mL
STABILITY	91 days (4 °C); 42 days (25 °C)
STABILITY REFERENCE	Nahata MC, et al. Am J Health Syst Pharm 1998; 55:1155-7
STORE	refrigerate
LABEL	shake well before use, refrigerate

INGREDIENT	STRENGTH	QUANTITY
Enalapril maleate tablets	10 mg	20
Deionized water		qs 200 mL

NOTE: In this study, the formulation was stored in plastic prescription bottles.

INSTRUCTIONS: Crush the tablets in a mortar and reduce to a fine powder. Add a small amount of water and levigate to a uniform paste. Add increasing amounts of water in geometric proportions, mix well, and make the suspension pourable. Transfer the suspension to a graduate. Rinse the mortar with water, transfer the rinsings to the graduate, and qs to 200 mL.

NOTES

GENERIC NAME	**Enalapril**
DOSAGE FORM	oral suspension
MADE FROM	tablets
CONCENTRATION	1 mg/mL
STABILITY	91 days
STABILITY REFERENCE	Nahata MC, et al. Am J Health Syst Pharm 1998; 55:1155-7
STORE	refrigerate (preferable) or at room temperature
LABEL	shake well before use, refrigerate

INGREDIENT	STRENGTH	QUANTITY
Enalapril maleate tablets	10 mg	20
Citric acid buffer solution (pH 5)		qs 200 mL

NOTE: In this study, the formulation was stored in plastic prescription bottles.

INSTRUCTIONS: Crush the tablets in a mortar and reduce to a fine powder. Add a small amount of the buffer solution and levigate to a uniform paste. Add increasing amounts of the buffer solution in geometric proportions, mix well, and make the suspension pourable. Transfer the suspension to a graduate. Rinse the mortar with the buffer solution, transfer the rinsings to the graduate, and qs to 200 mL.

NOTES

GENERIC NAME	**Enalapril**
DOSAGE FORM	oral suspension
MADE FROM	tablets
CONCENTRATION	1 mg/mL
STABILITY	60 days
STABILITY REFERENCE	Allen LV Jr, et al. Am J Health Syst Pharm 1998; 55:1915-20
STORE	refrigerate (preferable) or at room temperature
LABEL	shake well before use, refrigerate

INGREDIENT	STRENGTH	QUANTITY
Enalapril maleate tablets	20 mg	6
Cherry syrup (cherry syrup concentrate diluted 1:4 with simple syrup, NF)		qs 120 mL

NOTE: In this study, the formulation was stored in amber clear plastic (polyethylene terephthalate) prescription ovals.

INSTRUCTIONS: Crush the tablets and triturate to a fine powder. Add approximately 15 mL of vehicle and levigate to a uniform paste. Add vehicle in geometric proportions almost to volume, mix thoroughly, and transfer to a graduate. Rinse the mortar with vehicle, add to the graduate, and qs to 120 mL.

NOTES

GENERIC NAME	**Enalapril**
DOSAGE FORM	oral suspension
MADE FROM	tablets
CONCENTRATION	0.3 mg/mL
STABILITY	30 days
STABILITY REFERENCE	experience
STORE	refrigerate (preferred) or room temperature
LABEL	shake well before use, refrigerate

INGREDIENT	STRENGTH	QUANTITY
Enalapril	10 mg	3
Ora-Blend		qs 100 mL

INSTRUCTIONS: Triturate 3 tablets into a fine powder in a glass mortar. Wet the powder with a minimal quantity of Ora-Blend and levigate into a smooth suspension, adding the vehicle in geometric proportions. Continue adding the vehicle in geometric proportions with constant mixing. Transfer the suspension to a graduate. Rinse the mortar with sufficient vehicle and add to the graduate to bring the final volume to 100 mL.

NOTES

GENERIC NAME	**Ethacrynic Acid**
DOSAGE FORM	oral solution
MADE FROM	powder
CONCENTRATION	1 mg/mL
STABILITY	220 days
STABILITY REFERENCE	Gupta VD, et al. Am J Hosp Pharm 1978;35: 1382-5
STORE	room temperature
LABEL	room temperature

INGREDIENT	STRENGTH	QUANTITY
Ethacrynic acid powder		120 mg
Alcohol, USP		13 mL
[a]Parabens		
Sodium hydroxide	0.1N	qs to pH 7
Sorbitol solution	50%	qs ad 120 mL

[a]Methylparaben 0.005% and propylparaben 0.002% final concentration.

NOTE: Stability-indicating analytical methods not used.
INSTRUCTIONS: Mix ethacrynic acid powder, parabens, alcohol, and some of the sorbitol. Adjust pH to 7 with sodium hydroxide solution. Then qs with sorbitol solution, methylparaben 0.005%, and propylparaben 0.002% to final concentration.

NOTES

Ethambutol

GENERIC NAME	Ethambutol
DOSAGE FORM	oral suspension
MADE FROM	tablets
CONCENTRATION	50 mg/mL
STABILITY	30 days
STABILITY REFERENCE	experience
STORE	room temperature
LABEL	shake well before use, room temperature

INGREDIENT	STRENGTH	QUANTITY
Ethambutol tablets	400 mg	15
Cherry syrup, USP		qs 120 mL

INSTRUCTIONS: Remove coating from tablets with alcohol swabs. Triturate 15 tablets into a fine powder in a glass mortar. Wet the powder with minimal quantity of cherry syrup and levigate into a viscous smooth paste, adding the vehicle in geometric proportions. Continue adding the vehicle in geometric proportions with constant mixing. Transfer the suspension to a graduate. Rinse the mortar with sufficient vehicle and add to the graduate to bring the final volume to 120 mL. Mix well.

NOTES

Ethanol for Catheter Clearance

GENERIC NAME	
DOSAGE FORM	injection
MADE FROM	injection
CONCENTRATION	70%
STABILITY	1 year
STABILITY REFERENCE	experience, Pennington CR, et al. JPEN J Parenter Enteral Nutr 1987;11:507-8
STORE	refrigerate
LABEL	refrigerate

INGREDIENT	STRENGTH	QUANTITY
Ethanol injection	95%	25 mL
Sterile water for injection, USP		9 mL

NOTE: Stability-indicating analytical methods not used.
INSTRUCTIONS: Draw the ethanol into a 50-mL syringe. Add the water for injection to the syringe and mix thoroughly. Inject 5-mL aliquots into 10-mL vials and label.

NOTES

GENERIC NAME	**Ethinyl Estradiol**
DOSAGE FORM	solution
MADE FROM	powder
CONCENTRATION	1 mg/mL
STABILITY	4 years
STABILITY REFERENCE	personal communication (National Institutes of Health, 1987)
STORE	room temperature
LABEL	for compounding only

INGREDIENT	STRENGTH	QUANTITY
Ethinyl estradiol		100 mg
Absolute ethyl alcohol		100 mL

INSTRUCTIONS: Add powdered ethinyl estradiol to 90 mL of alcohol. Stir until dissolved, then qs to 100 mL with alcohol.

NOTES

Ethinyl Estradiol Diluting Fluid

GENERIC NAME	Ethinyl Estradiol Diluting Fluid
DOSAGE FORM	diluting fluid
MADE FROM	solution
STABILITY	46 months
STABILITY REFERENCE	personal communication (National Institutes of Health, 1987)
STORE	room temperature

INGREDIENT	STRENGTH	QUANTITY
Sodium benzoate		1 g
Absolute ethyl alcohol		5 mL
Purified water, USP		1000 mL

NOTE: Used to dilute ethinyl estradiol for treating Turner's syndrome.

INSTRUCTIONS: Dissolve sodium benzoate in water. Add alcohol and qs with water to 1 L. Adjust pH to 4 with 0.1N hydrochloric acid.

NOTES

GENERIC NAME	**Etoposide**
DOSAGE FORM	oral solution
MADE FROM	injection
CONCENTRATION	10 mg/mL
STABILITY	22 days
STABILITY REFERENCE	McLeod HL, et al. Am J Hosp Pharm 1992;49: 2784-5
STORE	room temperature

INGREDIENT	STRENGTH	QUANTITY
Etoposide injection	20 mg/mL (50-mL vials)	1
NaCl 0.9% injection		qs 100 mL

NOTE: In this study, the formulation was stored in 5-mL plastic oral syringes. Each mL of etoposide injection 20 mg/mL contains PEG 300 650 mg, ethyl alcohol 30.5% v/v, polysorbate 80 80 mg, benzyl alcohol 30 mg, citric acid 2 mg.

INSTRUCTIONS: Empty the contents of the vial in a 100-mL graduate and qs with NaCl 0.9% injection to 100 mL.

NOTES

GENERIC NAME	**Famotidine**
DOSAGE FORM	oral suspension
MADE FROM	tablets
CONCENTRATION	8 mg/mL
STABILITY	20 days (4 °C); 15 days (24 °C)
STABILITY REFERENCE	Quercia RA, et al. Am J Health Syst Pharm 1993; 50:691-3
STORE	refrigerate
LABEL	shake well before use, refrigerate

INGREDIENT	STRENGTH	QUANTITY
Famotidine tablets	40 mg	12
Distilled water		20 mL
Cherry syrup, USP		qs 60 mL

NOTE: In this study, the formulation was stored in amber glass bottles.
Commercially available as a powder for oral suspension (40 mg/5 mL) and chewable tablet (10 mg).

INSTRUCTIONS: Triturate twelve 40-mg famotidine tablets to a fine powder in a glass mortar. Add 10 mL of distilled water and levigate to a uniform paste. Add 30 mL of cherry syrup to the mortar in geometric proportions and transfer to a 100-mL graduate. Rinse the mortar with another 10 mL of distilled water and transfer to the graduate. Rinse the mortar with sufficient cherry syrup, add to the graduate, and qs to 60 mL.

NOTES

GENERIC NAME	**Famotidine**
DOSAGE FORM	oral suspension
MADE FROM	tablets
CONCENTRATION	8 mg/mL
STABILITY	95 days
STABILITY REFERENCE	Detinger PJ, et al. Am J Health Syst Pharm 2000; 57:1340-2
STORE	room temperature
LABEL	shake well before use

INGREDIENT	STRENGTH	QUANTITY
Famotidine tablets	40 mg	20
Sterile water for irrigation, USP		qs
Ora-Plus:Ora-Sweet	1:1	qs 100 mL

NOTE: In this study, the formulation was stored in amber polyethylene terephthalate bottles.

INSTRUCTIONS: Triturate twenty 40-mg famotidine tablets to a fine powder in a glass mortar. Add a sufficient amount of sterile water for irrigation, USP, and levigate to a uniform paste. Add approximately 30 mL of a 1:1 mixture of Ora-Plus and Ora-Sweet to the mortar in geometric proportions and transfer to a 100-mL graduate. Rinse the mortar with another 30 mL of the 1:1 mixture of Ora-Plus and Ora-Sweet and transfer to the graduate. Repeat and qs to 100 mL.

NOTES

GENERIC NAME	**Fentanyl**
DOSAGE FORM	nasal solution
MADE FROM	powder
CONCENTRATION	250 mcg/mL
STABILITY	30 days
STABILITY REFERENCE	Fentanyl 25 mcg/0.1 mL nasal spray. Int J Pharmaceut Compd 2000;4:57
STORE	protect from light
LABEL	for inhalation use only

INGREDIENT	STRENGTH	QUANTITY
Fentanyl citrate		3.9 mg (equivalent to 2.5 mg fentanyl)
Methylparabens		10 mg
Propylparabens		10 mg
Propylene glycol		0.2 mL
NaCl 0.9% for inhalation		qs 10 mL

NOTE: Stability-indicating analytical methods not used. Based on *United States Pharmacopeia National Formulary* (Rockville, MD: US Pharmacopeial Convention) beyond-use date recommendation in the absence of stability information.

INSTRUCTIONS: Dissolve the parabens in propylene glycol and the fentanyl in 9 mL of the NaCl 0.9% solution. Mix the two solutions in geometric proportions. Add sufficient NaCl 0.9% solution to qs to 10 mL and mix. Filter through a 0.2-μm filter and store in a sterile metered-spray bottle.

NOTES

GENERIC NAME	# Flecainide
DOSAGE FORM	oral suspension
MADE FROM	tablets
CONCENTRATION	20 mg/mL
STABILITY	60 days
STABILITY REFERENCE	Allen LV Jr, et al. Am J Health Syst Pharm 1996; 53:2179-84
STORE	refrigerate (preferable) or at room temperature
LABEL	shake well before use, refrigerate

INGREDIENT	STRENGTH	QUANTITY
Flecainide acetate tablets	100 mg	24
Ora-Plus:Ora-Sweet or Ora-Plus:Ora-Sweet SF	1:1 mixture	qs 120 mL

NOTE: In this study, the formulation was stored in amber clear plastic (polyethylene terephthalate) prescription ovals.

INSTRUCTIONS: Crush the tablets and triturate to a fine powder. Add approximately 20 mL of vehicle and levigate to a uniform paste. Add vehicle in geometric proportions almost to volume, mix thoroughly, and transfer to a graduate. Rinse the mortar with vehicle, add to the graduate, and qs to 120 mL.

NOTES

GENERIC NAME	**Flecainide**
DOSAGE FORM	oral suspension
MADE FROM	tablets
CONCENTRATION	20 mg/mL
STABILITY	60 days
STABILITY REFERENCE	Allen LV Jr, et al. Am J Health Syst Pharm 1996;53:2179-84
STORE	refrigerate (preferable) or at room temperature
LABEL	shake well before use, refrigerate

INGREDIENT	STRENGTH	QUANTITY
Flecainide acetate tablets	100 mg	24
Cherry syrup (cherry syrup concentrate diluted 1:4 with simple syrup, NF)		qs 120 mL

NOTE: In this study, the formulation was stored in amber clear plastic (polyethylene terephthalate) prescription ovals.

INSTRUCTIONS: Crush the tablets and triturate to a fine powder. Add approximately 20 mL of vehicle and levigate to a uniform paste. Add vehicle in geometric proportions almost to volume, mix thoroughly, and transfer to a graduate. Rinse the mortar with vehicle, add to the graduate, and qs to 120 mL.

NOTES

GENERIC NAME	**Fluconazole**
DOSAGE FORM	oral liquid
MADE FROM	tablets
CONCENTRATION	1 mg/mL
STABILITY	15 days
STABILITY REFERENCE	Yamreudeewong W, et al. Am J Hosp Pharm 1993;50:2366-7
STORE	refrigerate (preferable) or at room temperature
LABEL	shake well before use, refrigerate

INGREDIENT	STRENGTH	QUANTITY
Fluconazole tablets	100 mg	5
Water, deionized		qs 500 mL

NOTE: In this study, the formulation was stored in borosilicate glass vials with teflon septa. Commercially available as an oral suspension, 10 mg/mL and 40 mg/mL.

INSTRUCTIONS: Pulverize the tablets in a mortar and add water to make a suspension. Transfer the suspension to a graduate and qs with water to final desired volume.

NOTES

GENERIC NAME	**Flucytosine**
DOSAGE FORM	oral suspension
MADE FROM	capsules
CONCENTRATION	10 mg/mL
STABILITY	60 days
STABILITY REFERENCE	Allen LV Jr, et al. Am J Health Syst Pharm 1996;53:1944-9
STORE	refrigerate (preferable) or at room temperature
LABEL	shake well before use, refrigerate

INGREDIENT	STRENGTH	QUANTITY
Flucytosine capsules	250 mg	4
Ora-Plus:Ora-Sweet	1:1	
or Ora-Plus:Ora-Sweet SF		qs 100 mL

NOTE: In this study, the formulation was stored in amber clear plastic (polyethylene terephthalate) prescription ovals.

INSTRUCTIONS: Triturate the contents of the capsules in a mortar. Add approximately 10 mL of vehicle and levigate to a uniform paste. Add vehicle in geometric proportions almost to volume, mix thoroughly, and transfer to a graduate. Rinse the mortar with vehicle, add to the graduate, and qs to 100 mL.

NOTES

GENERIC NAME	**Flucytosine**
DOSAGE FORM	oral suspension
MADE FROM	capsules
CONCENTRATION	10 mg/mL
STABILITY	60 days
STABILITY REFERENCE	Allen LV Jr, et al. Am J Health Syst Pharm 1996;53:1944-9
STORE	refrigerate (preferable) or at room temperature
LABEL	shake well before use, refrigerate

INGREDIENT	STRENGTH	QUANTITY
Flucytosine capsules	250 mg	4
Cherry syrup (cherry syrup concentrate diluted 1:4 with simple syrup, NF)		qs 100 mL

NOTE: In this study, the formulation was stored in amber clear plastic (polyethylene terephthalate) prescription ovals.

INSTRUCTIONS: Triturate the contents of the capsules in a mortar. Add approximately 10 mL of vehicle and levigate to a uniform paste. Add vehicle in geometric proportions almost to volume, mix thoroughly, and transfer to a graduate. Rinse the mortar with vehicle, add to the graduate, and qs to 100 mL.

NOTES

GENERIC NAME	**Flucytosine**
DOSAGE FORM	oral suspension
MADE FROM	capsules
CONCENTRATION	10 mg/mL
STABILITY	70 days
STABILITY REFERENCE	Wintermeyer SM, et al. Am J Health Syst Pharm 1996;53:407-9
STORE	refrigerate (preferable) or at room temperature
LABEL	shake well before use, refrigerate

INGREDIENT	STRENGTH	QUANTITY
Flucytosine capsules	500 mg	2
Purified water, USP		qs 100 mL

NOTE: In this study, the formulation was stored in glass or plastic prescription bottles.

INSTRUCTIONS: Empty the contents of capsules into a glass mortar and levigate with a small amount of water into a smooth paste. Add more water in geometric proportions, mixing well, and transfer to a graduate. Rinse the mortar repeatedly with purified water, add to the graduate, and qs to 100 mL.

NOTES

GENERIC NAME	**Flucytosine**
DOSAGE FORM	oral suspension
MADE FROM	capsules
CONCENTRATION	50 mg/mL
STABILITY	90 days
STABILITY REFERENCE	VandenBussche HL, et al. Am J Health Syst Pharm 2002;59:1853-5
STORE	refrigerate (preferable) or room temperature
LABEL	shake well before use, refrigerate

INGREDIENT	STRENGTH	QUANTITY
Flucytosine capsules	500 mg	6
Ora-Plus		30 mL
Simple syrup, NF		101 mL
Strawberry fountain syrup		19 mL

NOTE: In this study, the formulation was stored in amber child-resistant prescription bottles.

INSTRUCTIONS: Prepare strawberry syrup by mixing simple syrup, NF, and strawberry fountain syrup in geometric proportions with constant stirring. Triturate the contents of 6 capsules into a fine powder in a glass mortar. Mix equal quantities of Ora-Plus and strawberry syrup (initially prepared) in geometric proportions, with constant stirring, to produce 60 mL. Using 15 mL of this mixture, levigate the powder into a smooth suspension, adding the vehicle in geometric proportions. Transfer the suspension to a 2-oz child-resistant amber prescription bottle. Rinse the mortar with sufficient vehicle into the bottle to bring the final volume in the bottle to 60 mL.

NOTES

GENERIC NAME	**Flucytosine**
DOSAGE FORM	oral suspension
MADE FROM	capsules
CONCENTRATION	50 mg/mL
STABILITY	90 days
STABILITY REFERENCE	VandenBussche HL, et al. Am J Health Syst Pharm 2002;59:1853-5
STORE	refrigerate (preferable) or room temperature
LABEL	shake well before use, refrigerate

INGREDIENT	STRENGTH	QUANTITY
Flucytosine capsules	500 mg	6
Ora-Plus		30 mL
Ora-Sweet SF		30 mL

NOTE: In this study, the formulation was stored in amber child-resistant prescription bottles.

INSTRUCTIONS: Triturate the contents of 6 capsules into a fine powder in a glass mortar. Mix equal quantities of Ora-Plus and Ora-Sweet SF in geometric proportions with constant stirring to produce 60 mL. Using 15 mL of this mixture, levigate the powder into a smooth suspension, adding the vehicle in geometric proportions. Transfer the suspension to a 2-oz child-resistant amber prescription bottle. Rinse the mortar with sufficient vehicle into the bottle to bring the final volume in the bottle to 60 mL.

NOTES

GENERIC NAME	**Fludrocortisone**
DOSAGE FORM	oral suspension
MADE FROM	tablets
CONCENTRATION	any concentration
STABILITY	14 days
STABILITY REFERENCE	Woods DJ. www.pharminfotech.co.nz/emixt
STORE	refrigerate
LABEL	shake well before use, refrigerate

INGREDIENT	STRENGTH	QUANTITY
Fludrocortisone acetate tablets		qs
Sodium carboxymethyl-cellulose	1 g	
Syrup		10 mL
[a]Parabens	0.1%	
Citric acid monohydrate	600 mg	
Lemon spirit (optional)		0.25 mL
Water		qs 100 mL

[a]Methyl hydroxybenzoate 4 g, propyl hydroxybenzoate 1 g, propylene glycol qs 100 mL. Mix 2 mL of this solution with 100 mL of formulation to produce parabens 0.1%.

NOTE: If available, 0.5 mL of polysorbate 80 can be used to wet the crushed tablets. Alternatively, use ethanol. In this study, the formulation was stored in amber glass bottles. Stability-indicating analytical methods not used.

INSTRUCTIONS: In a glass mortar, levigate carboxymethylcellulose with sufficient amount (5–10 mL) of water to form a uniform paste. Add approximately 40 mL of water to the paste in geometric proportions with vigorous levigation (preferably use a blender). Transfer the suspension to a suitable container for heating. Heat the dispersion to about 60 °C, with moderate stirring, until the carboxymethylcellulose dissolves. Allow to cool and stand for 1–2 hours to form a clear gel. Crush the tablets and triturate to a fine powder in the glass mortar. Add 0.5 mL of polysorbate 80 and levigate to a uniform paste. Add carboxymethylcellulose gel in geometric proportions and mix well. Dissolve citric acid in approximately 5 mL of water. Add syrup, the parabens solution, and the citric acid solution in geometric proportions and mix well. Add the lemon flavor and mix. Transfer to a graduate, rinse the mortar with water, add to the graduate, and qs to 100 mL.

NOTES

GENERIC NAME	**Fluoxetine**
DOSAGE FORM	oral solution
MADE FROM	solution
CONCENTRATION	1 mg/mL
STABILITY	56 days (5 °C and 30 °C)
STABILITY REFERENCE	Peterson JA, et al. Am J Hosp Pharm 1994;51:1342-5
STORE	refrigerate (preferable) or at room temperature
LABEL	refrigerate

INGREDIENT	STRENGTH	QUANTITY
Fluoxetine solution	4 mg/mL	5 mL
Simple syrup, NF		15 mL

NOTE: In this study, the formulation was stored in amber glass bottles. Commercially available as a solution, 20 mg/5 mL.

INSTRUCTIONS: Measure the two liquids in graduates and mix thoroughly in geometric proportions.

NOTES

GENERIC NAME	**Fluoxetine**
DOSAGE FORM	oral solution
MADE FROM	solution
CONCENTRATION	2 mg/mL
STABILITY	56 days
STABILITY REFERENCE	Peterson JA, et al. Am J Hosp Pharm 1994;51: 1342-5
STORE	refrigerate (preferable) or at room temperature
LABEL	refrigerate

INGREDIENT	STRENGTH	QUANTITY
Fluoxetine solution	4 mg/mL	10 mL
Simple syrup, NF		10 mL

NOTE: In this study, the formulation was stored in amber glass bottles. Commercially available as a solution, 20 mg/5 mL.

INSTRUCTIONS: Measure the two liquids in graduates and mix thoroughly in geometric proportions.

NOTES

GENERIC NAME	**Folic Acid**
DOSAGE FORM	oral solution
MADE FROM	injection
CONCENTRATION	0.05 mg/mL
STABILITY	30 days
STABILITY REFERENCE	Smith SG. Pharm J 1976;216:108
STORE	room temperature

INGREDIENT	STRENGTH	QUANTITY
Folic acid injection	5 mg/mL	1 mL
Sodium hydroxide	0.1N	2.8 mL
Purified water, USP		qs ad 100 mL

NOTE: The study included Nipa esters as preservative; however, no concentration was provided.

INSTRUCTIONS: Mix the folic acid and 90 mL of water. Adjust pH to 8–8.5 with sodium hydroxide, then qs to volume with water.

NOTES

GENERIC NAME	**Fumagillin**
DOSAGE FORM	ophthalmic solution
MADE FROM	crystals
CONCENTRATION	70 mcg/mL
STABILITY	14 days
STABILITY REFERENCE	Abdel-Rahman SM, et al. Am J Health Syst Pharm 1999;56:547-50
STORE	refrigerate
LABEL	refrigerate, for ophthalmic use only

INGREDIENT	STRENGTH	QUANTITY
[a]Fumagillin crystals		120 mg
NaCl 0.9% injection, USP		20 mL
Dacriose		20 mL

[a]Fumagillin bicyclohexylammonium crystals

NOTE: Sterility testing performed.
INSTRUCTIONS: Weigh 120 mg of fumagillin bicyclohexylammonium crystals and place in a clean amber plastic vial. Add 10 mL of NaCl 0.9% injection, USP, to the vial and mix to dissolve. Draw this solution into a 60-mL sterile syringe. Rinse the vial with 10 mL of NaCl 0.9% solution and draw into same syringe. Draw an additional 40 mL of ophthalmic irrigating solution into the same syringe and mix by shaking. Filter the resulting solution through a 0.22-μm filter into sterile dropper bottles and label.

NOTES

GENERIC NAME	**Furosemide**
DOSAGE FORM	oral liquid
MADE FROM	injection
CONCENTRATION	1 mg/mL
STABILITY	30 days
STABILITY REFERENCE	Ghanekar AG, et al. J Pharmaceut Sci 1978;67: 808-11
STORE	room temperature

INGREDIENT	STRENGTH	QUANTITY
Furosemide injection	10 mg/mL	10 mL
Syrpalta		qs 100 mL

NOTE: Commercially available as an oral solution, 10 mg/mL and 40 mg/5 mL.

INSTRUCTIONS: Mix furosemide injection and the vehicle in geometric proportions, then qs with vehicle to 100 mL.

NOTES

GENERIC NAME	**Furosemide**
DOSAGE FORM	oral liquid
MADE FROM	injection
CONCENTRATION	2 mg/mL
STABILITY	30 days
STABILITY REFERENCE	Ghanekar AG, et al. J Pharmaceut Sci 1978;67: 808-11
STORE	room temperature

INGREDIENT	STRENGTH	QUANTITY
Furosemide injection	10 mg/mL	10 mL
Syrpalta		qs 50 mL

NOTE:	Commercially available as an oral solution, 10 mg/mL and 40 mg/5 mL.
INSTRUCTIONS:	Mix furosemide injection and the vehicle in geometric proportions, then qs with vehicle to 50 mL.

NOTES

GENERIC NAME	**Gabapentin**
DOSAGE FORM	oral suspension
MADE FROM	capsules
CONCENTRATION	100 mg/mL
STABILITY	91 days (4 °C); 56 days (25 °C)
STABILITY REFERENCE	Nahata MC. Pediatr Neurol 1999;20:195-7
STORE	refrigerate
LABEL	shake well before use, refrigerate

INGREDIENT	STRENGTH	QUANTITY
Gabapentin capsules	300 mg	20
Simple syrup, NF		
Methylcellulose	1%	aa qs 60 mL

NOTE: In this study, the formulation was stored in amber plastic prescription bottles.

INSTRUCTIONS: Empty the capsules into a mortar and mix with a small amount of syrup until a smooth paste is formed; qs with the remaining syrup in small quantities while mixing. Transfer the mixture to a graduate and qs with methylcellulose.

NOTES

GENERIC NAME	**Gabapentin**
DOSAGE FORM	oral suspension
MADE FROM	capsules
CONCENTRATION	100 mg/mL
STABILITY	91 days (4 °C); 56 days (25 °C)
STABILITY REFERENCE	Nahata MC. Pediatr Neurol 1999;20:195-7
STORE	refrigerate
LABEL	shake well before use, refrigerate

INGREDIENT	STRENGTH	QUANTITY
Gabapentin capsules	300 mg	20
Ora-Plus		
Ora-Sweet		aa qs 60 mL

NOTE: In this study, the formulation was stored in amber plastic prescription bottles.

INSTRUCTIONS: Empty the capsules into a mortar. Mix the two vehicles together. Add a small amount of the mixture to the powder and mix until a smooth paste is formed; qs with the remaining mixture in small quantities while mixing.

NOTES

GENERIC NAME	**Ganciclovir**
DOSAGE FORM	oral suspension
MADE FROM	capsules
CONCENTRATION	100 mg/mL
STABILITY	123 days
STABILITY REFERENCE	Anaizi NH, et al. Am J Health Syst Pharm 1999; 56:1738-41
STORE	room temperature
LABEL	shake well before use

INGREDIENT	STRENGTH	QUANTITY
Ganciclovir capsules	250 mg	80
Ora-Sweet or Ora-Sweet SF		qs ad 200 mL

NOTE: In this study, the formulation was stored in amber plastic (polyethylene terephthalate) bottles.

INSTRUCTIONS: Empty the contents of the capsules into a mortar and reduce to a fine powder. Avoid contact with drug. Add a small amount of vehicle and mix to a uniform paste. Add 50 mL of vehicle while mixing and transfer to a graduate. Rinse the mortar with vehicle and add to the graduate. Then qs to 200 mL with vehicle, mix well, and place in an amber Rx bottle.

NOTES

Gentamicin Sulfate, Fortified

GENERIC NAME	
DOSAGE FORM	ophthalmic drops
MADE FROM	injection
CONCENTRATION	8 mg/mL
STABILITY	14 days
STABILITY REFERENCE	Doughman DJ. Clinical ophthalmology. Vol. 4. Philadelphia: Harper & Row, 1982:1-19
STORE	refrigerate
LABEL	refrigerate; for ophthalmic use only

INGREDIENT	STRENGTH	QUANTITY
Gentamicin injection	40 mg/mL	0.78 mL
Gentamicin ophthalmic drops	3 mg/mL	5 mL

NOTE: For special ophthalmic procedures.
INSTRUCTIONS: Add the gentamicin injection to the bottle of gentamicin ophthalmic drops.

NOTES

GENERIC NAME	**Gentamicin Sulfate, Fortified**
DOSAGE FORM	ophthalmic drops
MADE FROM	injection
CONCENTRATION	13.6 mg/mL
STABILITY	90 days (4–8 °C)
STABILITY REFERENCE	McBride HA, et al. Am J Hosp Pharm 1991;48: 507-8
STORE	refrigerate
LABEL	refrigerate; for ophthalmic use only

INGREDIENT	STRENGTH	QUANTITY
Gentamicin sulfate ophthalmic solution (Genoptic)	3 mg/mL	5 mL
Gentamicin sulfate injection	40 mg/mL	2 mL

NOTE: Sterility testing not performed.

INSTRUCTIONS: Add 2 mL of 40-mg/mL injectable solution to 5 mL of 3-mg/mL ophthalmic solution using aseptic technique and a laminar air flow hood. American Society of Health-System Pharmacists' guidelines (Am J Hosp Pharm 1993;50:1462-3) for compounding ophthalmic products should be considered while preparing this formulation.

NOTES

GENERIC NAME	**Glutamine**
DOSAGE FORM	oral suspension
MADE FROM	powder
CONCENTRATION	500 mg/mL
STABILITY	30 days
STABILITY REFERENCE	experience
STORE	refrigerate
LABEL	shake well before use, refrigerate

INGREDIENT	STRENGTH	QUANTITY
Glutamine powder		30 g
Ora-Plus		9 mL
Ora-Sweet		18 mL
Sterile water for irrigation		9 mL

NOTE: In this study, the formulation was stored in amber prescription bottle.

INSTRUCTIONS: Triturate glutamine into a fine powder in a glass mortar. Mix Ora-Plus, Ora-Sweet, and sterile water for irrigation in 1:1:2 proportion to prepare the base vehicle. Wet the powder with a minimal quantity of the vehicle and levigate into a viscous smooth paste, adding the vehicle in geometric proportions. Continue adding the vehicle in geometric proportions with constant mixing to. Transfer the suspension to a graduate. Rinse the mortar with sufficient vehicle and add to the graduate to bring the final volume to 60 mL. Mix well.

NOTES

GENERIC NAME	**Glycine (aminoacetic acid)**
DOSAGE FORM	oral solution
MADE FROM	powder
CONCENTRATION	2.25%
STABILITY	180 days
STABILITY REFERENCE	experience
STORE	refrigerate
LABEL	refrigerate

INGREDIENT	STRENGTH	QUANTITY
Glycine powder		2.25 g
Distilled water		qs 100 mL

INSTRUCTIONS: Triturate glycine into a fine powder in a glass mortar. Dissolve the powder in water. Transfer the solution to a graduate. Rinse the mortar with sufficient water and add to the graduate to bring the final volume to 100 mL. Stir well.

NOTES

GENERIC NAME	**Glycopyrrolate**
DOSAGE FORM	oral suspension
MADE FROM	tablets
CONCENTRATION	0.2 mg/mL
STABILITY	14 days
STABILITY REFERENCE	Nahata MC, et al. Presented at: American Society of Health-System Pharmacists Midyear Clinical Meeting, December 2004 (poster)
STORE	refrigerate (preferable) or room temperature
LABEL	refrigerate, shake well before use

INGREDIENT	STRENGTH	QUANTITY
Glycopyrrolate tablets	1 mg	24
Simple syrup NF: 1% methylcellulose suspension	1:10	qs 120 mL

NOTE: This formulation was stored in amber prescription bottles.

INSTRUCTIONS: Mix simple syrup and 1% methylcellulose suspension together thoroughly in a glass mortar pestle, in geometric proportions, to prepare the vehicle. Triturate the tablets into a fine powder and levigate with small proportion of the vehicle into a smooth suspension. Add vehicle in geometric proportions with constant mixing. Transfer to a graduate. Rinse the mortar and pestle with sufficient vehicle and transfer to graduate to make up the final volume.

NOTES

GENERIC NAME	**Glycopyrrolate**
DOSAGE FORM	oral suspension
MADE FROM	tablets
CONCENTRATION	0.2 mg/mL
STABILITY	14 days
STABILITY REFERENCE	Nahata MC, et al. Presented at: American Society of Health-System Pharmacists Midyear Clinical Meeting, December 2004 (poster)
STORE	refrigerate (preferable) or room temperature
LABEL	refrigerate, shake well before use

INGREDIENT	STRENGTH	QUANTITY
Glycopyrrolate tablets	1 mg	24
Ora-Plus:Ora-Sweet	1:1	qs 120 mL

NOTE: This formulation was stored in amber prescription bottles.

INSTRUCTIONS: Mix Ora-Plus and Ora-Sweet together thoroughly in a glass mortar pestle, in geometric proportions, to prepare the vehicle. Triturate the tablets into a fine powder and levigate with small proportion of the vehicle into a smooth suspension. Add vehicle in geometric proportions, with constant mixing. Transfer to a graduate. Rinse the mortar and pestle with sufficient vehicle and transfer to graduate to make up the final volume.

NOTES

GENERIC NAME	**Granisetron**
DOSAGE FORM	oral suspension
MADE FROM	tablets
CONCENTRATION	0.05 mg/mL
STABILITY	91 days
STABILITY REFERENCE	Nahata MC, et al. Am J Health Syst Pharm 1998;55:2511-3
STORE	refrigerate (preferable) or at room temperature
LABEL	shake well before use, refrigerate

INGREDIENT	STRENGTH	QUANTITY
Granisetron hydrochloride tablet	1 mg	1
Methylcellulose	1%	
Simple syrup, NF		aa qs 20 mL

NOTE: In this study, the formulation was stored in amber plastic prescription bottles.

INSTRUCTIONS: Crush the tablets in a mortar. Mix the two vehicles together. Add the vehicle mixture to the powder in small amounts while mixing. Transfer to a graduate and qs with vehicle mixture.

NOTES

GENERIC NAME	**Granisetron**
DOSAGE FORM	oral suspension
MADE FROM	tablets
CONCENTRATION	0.05 mg/mL
STABILITY	91 days
STABILITY REFERENCE	Nahata MC, et al. Am J Health Syst Pharm 1998;55:2511-3
STORE	refrigerate (preferable) or at room temperature
LABEL	shake well before use, refrigerate

INGREDIENT	STRENGTH	QUANTITY
Granisetron hydrochloride tablet	1 mg	1
Ora-Sweet:Ora-Plus		aa qs 20 mL

NOTE: In this study, the formulation was stored in amber plastic prescription bottles.

INSTRUCTIONS: Crush the tablets in a mortar. Mix the two vehicles together. Add the vehicle mixture to the powder in small amounts while mixing. Transfer to a graduate and qs with vehicle mixture.

NOTES

GENERIC NAME	**Granisetron**
DOSAGE FORM	oral suspension
MADE FROM	tablets
CONCENTRATION	0.2 mg/mL
STABILITY	14 days
STABILITY REFERENCE	Quercia RA, et al. Am J Health Syst Pharm 1997;54:1404-6
STORE	refrigerate (preferable) or at room temperature
LABEL	shake well before use, refrigerate

INGREDIENT	STRENGTH	QUANTITY
Granisetron hydrochloride tablets	1 mg	12
Distilled water		30 mL
Cherry syrup		qs 60 mL

NOTE: In this study, the formulation was stored in amber plastic prescription bottles.

INSTRUCTIONS: Crush twelve 1-mg granisetron tablets into a fine powder. Levigate with 30 mL of distilled water added in geometric proportions. Transfer the contents to a 100-mL graduate. Rinse the mortar with 10 mL of cherry syrup and transfer to the graduate. Repeat with a sufficient quantity of cherry syrup and qs volume to 60 mL.

NOTES

GENERIC NAME	**Griseofulvin**
DOSAGE FORM	oral suspension
MADE FROM	tablets
CONCENTRATION	any required concentration
STABILITY	15 days
STABILITY REFERENCE	Woods DJ. www.pharminfotech.co.nz/emixt
STORE	refrigerate (preferable) or at room temperature
LABEL	shake well before use, refrigerate, protect from light

INGREDIENT	STRENGTH	QUANTITY
[a]Griseofulvin hydrochloride tablets		qs
Ethanol		1 mL
Propylene glycol (if available)		5 mL
[b]Parabens	0.1%	
Methylcellulose	1%	50 mL
Water		qs 100 mL

[a]Use ultramicrosize griseofulvin tablets if available, as this form has a more consistent bioavailability.
[b]Methyl hydroxybenzoate 4 g, propyl hydroxybenzoate 1 g, propylene glycol qs 100 mL. Mix 2 mL of this solution to 100 mL of formulation to give parabens 0.1%.

NOTE:	Stability-indicating analytical methods not used. Commercially available as an oral suspension, 125 mg/5 mL, and contains alcohol 0.2%.
INSTRUCTIONS:	Crush the tablets and triturate to a fine powder. Levigate the powder with propylene glycol into a uniform paste. Add the methylcellulose solution in geometric proportions and mix well. Add the parabens solution and alcohol and mix. Transfer to a graduate, rinse the mortar with water, add to the graduate, and qs to 100 mL.

NOTES

GENERIC NAME	**Hydralazine**
DOSAGE FORM	injection
MADE FROM	injection
CONCENTRATION	2 mg/mL
STABILITY	24 hours
STABILITY REFERENCE	experience
STORE	room temperature, store in an empty sterile vial

INGREDIENT	STRENGTH	QUANTITY
Hydralazine hydrochloride injection	20 mg/mL	1 mL
Bacteriostatic water for injection		9 mL

INSTRUCTIONS: Mix the ingredients in a syringe aseptically.

NOTES

GENERIC NAME	**Hydralazine**
DOSAGE FORM	oral solution
MADE FROM	powder
CONCENTRATION	1 mg/mL
STABILITY	30 days
STABILITY REFERENCE	Hydralazine hydrochloride oral solution. United States Pharmacopeia XXIII/National Formulary 18. Supplement 9. November 1998:4556
STORE	refrigerate, in light-resistant plastic or glass bottle
LABEL	refrigerate, protect from light

INGREDIENT	STRENGTH	QUANTITY
Hydralazine hydrochloride		100 mg
Sorbitol solution 70%		40 g
Methylparabens		65 mg
Propylparabens		35 mg
Propylene glycol		10 g
Aspartame		50 mg
Purified water		qs 100 mL

NOTE: May mix appropriate dose with fruit juice or applesauce just prior to administration.

INSTRUCTIONS: Dissolve hydralazine hydrochloride in 30 mL of purified water, add the aspartame, and shake or stir until the solids have dissolved. Add the sorbitol solution. In a separate container, dissolve an aliquot portion of an intimate homogenous mixture of accurately weighed quantities of methylparabens and propylparabens in the propylene glycol and, while stirring, add this mixture to the solution containing the hydralazine hydrochloride. Add sufficient water to make the product measure 100 mL and mix.

NOTES

GENERIC NAME	**Hydralazine**
DOSAGE FORM	oral solution
MADE FROM	powder
CONCENTRATION	10 mg/mL
STABILITY	30 days
STABILITY REFERENCE	Hydralazine hydrochloride oral solution. United States Pharmacopeia XXIII/National Formulary 18. Supplement 9. November 1998:4556
STORE	refrigerate, in light-resistant plastic or glass bottle
LABEL	refrigerate

INGREDIENT	STRENGTH	QUANTITY
Hydralazine hydrochloride		1.0 g
Sorbitol solution 70%		40 g
Methylparaben		65 mg
Propylparaben		35 mg
Propylene glycol		10 g
Aspartame		50 mg
Purified water, USP		qs 100 mL

NOTE: May mix appropriate dose with fruit juice or applesauce just prior to administration.

INSTRUCTIONS: Dissolve hydralazine hydrochloride in 30 mL of purified water, add the aspartame, and shake or stir until the solids have dissolved. Add the sorbitol solution. In a separate container, dissolve an aliquot portion of an intimate homogenous mixture of accurately weighed quantities of methylparabens and propylparabens in the propylene glycol and, while stirring, add this mixture to the solution containing the hydralazine hydrochloride. Add sufficient water to make the product measure 100 mL and mix.

NOTES

GENERIC NAME	**Hydralazine**
DOSAGE FORM	oral suspension
MADE FROM	tablets
CONCENTRATION	4 mg/mL
STABILITY	1 day
STABILITY REFERENCE	Allen LV Jr, et al. Am J Health Syst Pharm 1998;55:1915-20
STORE	refrigerate
LABEL	shake well before use, refrigerate

INGREDIENT	STRENGTH	QUANTITY
Hydralazine tablets	100 mg	4
Ora-Plus		
Ora-Sweet		aa qs 100 mL

NOTE: In this study, the formulation was stored in amber clear polyethylene terephthalate prescription ovals.

INSTRUCTIONS: Crush the tablets in a mortar to a fine powder. Levigate with approximately 15 mL of 1:1 mixture of Ora-Plus and Ora-Sweet to a uniform paste. Add the vehicle in geometric proportions almost to volume. Transfer the contents to a graduate, rinse mortar with more vehicle, and add to graduate to qs to 100 mL.

NOTES

GENERIC NAME	**Hydralazine**
DOSAGE FORM	oral suspension
MADE FROM	tablets
CONCENTRATION	4 mg/mL
STABILITY	2 days
STABILITY REFERENCE	Allen LV Jr, et al. Am J Health Syst Pharm 1998;55:1915-20
STORE	refrigerate
LABEL	shake well before use, refrigerate

INGREDIENT	STRENGTH	QUANTITY
Hydralazine tablets	100 mg	4
Ora-Plus		
Ora-Sweet SF		aa qs 100 mL

NOTE: In this study, the formulation was stored in amber clear polyethylene terephthalate prescription ovals.

INSTRUCTIONS: Crush the tablets in a mortar to a fine powder. Levigate with approximately 15 mL of 1:1 mixture of Ora-Plus and Ora-Sweet SF to a uniform paste. Add the vehicle in geometric proportions almost to volume. Transfer the contents to a graduate, rinse mortar with more vehicle, and add to graduate to qs to 100 mL.

NOTES

Hydrochloric Acid 0.1 Normal

GENERIC NAME	
DOSAGE FORM	catheter clearance injection
MADE FROM	37% hydrochloric acid
CONCENTRATION	0.1 N
STABILITY	6 months
STABILITY REFERENCE	experience, Shulman RJ, et al. JPEN J Parenter Enteral Nutr 1988;12:509-10, Duffy LF, et al. J Pediatr 1989;114:1002-4
STORE	glass

INGREDIENT	STRENGTH	QUANTITY
Hydrochloric acid	37%	8.3 mL
Bacteriostatic water for injection		1000 mL

NOTE: Stability-indicating analytical methods not used.

INSTRUCTIONS: Transfer the hydrochloric acid from the original container to a clean glass beaker with caution. Draw 8.3 mL of hydrochloric acid into a glass syringe and add to a 1-L bag of water for injection. Mix well. Transfer from the bag into a sterile 10-mL vial through a 0.22-μm Millipore filter and syringe setup.

NOTES

GENERIC NAME	# Hydrochlorothiazide
DOSAGE FORM	oral suspension
MADE FROM	tablets
CONCENTRATION	5 mg/mL
STABILITY	60 days
STABILITY REFERENCE	experience, Allen LV Jr, et al. Am J Health Syst Pharm 1996;53:2304-8
STORE	room temperature
LABEL	shake well before use

INGREDIENT	STRENGTH	QUANTITY
Hydrochlorothiazide tablets	50 mg	10
Ora-Blend		qs 100 mL

NOTE: Store in a glass amber bottle.

INSTRUCTIONS: Triturate the tablets into a fine powder in a glass mortar. Levigate the powder with a small portion of the vehicle into a smooth suspension. Add vehicle in geometric proportions, with constant mixing. Transfer the suspension to a graduate. Rinse the mortar with sufficient vehicle and add to the graduate to bring the final volume to 100 mL.

NOTES

GENERIC NAME	**Hydrocortisone**
DOSAGE FORM	oral suspension
MADE FROM	tablets
CONCENTRATION	2.5 mg/mL
STABILITY	30 days
STABILITY REFERENCE	Fawcett JP, et al. Ann Pharmacother 1995;29: 987-90
STORE	refrigerate (preferable) or at room temperature
LABEL	shake well before use, refrigerate

INGREDIENT	STRENGTH	QUANTITY
Hydrocortisone base tablets	20 mg	12.5
[a]Polysorbate 80		0.5 mL
[b]Sodium carboxymethylcellulose	1 g	
Methyl hydroxybenzoate	0.02 g	
Propyl hydroxybenzoate	0.08 g	
Syrup BP		10 mL
Citric acid monohydrate	0.600 g	
Water		qs 100 mL

[a]Polysorbate 80 helps to wet the hydrocortisone.
[b]Use methylcellulose 1% as an alternative.

NOTE:	In this study, the formulation was stored in amber high-density polyethylene containers.
INSTRUCTIONS:	Dissolve methyl hydroxybenzoate, propyl hydroxybenzoate, citric acid, and syrup BP in hot water. Cool this solution. Triturate sodium carboxymethylcellulose with this solution, allowing to stand overnight. This is your vehicle. Crush and triturate the tablets in a glass mortar, wet with polysorbate 80, and levigate to a uniform paste. Add the vehicle in geometric proportions, mix well, and transfer to a graduate. Rinse the mortar with the vehicle, transferring to the graduate to qs to 100 mL.

NOTES

GENERIC NAME	**Hydrocortisone**
DOSAGE FORM	oral suspension
MADE FROM	tablets
CONCENTRATION	2 mg/mL
STABILITY	60 days
STABILITY REFERENCE	Chong G, et al. J Inform Pharmacother 2003; 13:100-10
STORE	refrigerate (preferable) or room temperature
LABEL	refrigerate, shake well before use,

INGREDIENT	STRENGTH	QUANTITY
Hydrocortisone tablets	20 mg	10
Ora-Blend		qs 100 mL

INSTRUCTIONS: Triturate the tablets into a fine powder in a glass mortar. Levigate the powder with a small portion of the vehicle into a smooth suspension. Add vehicle in geometric proportions, with constant mixing. Transfer the suspension to a graduate. Rinse the mortar with sufficient vehicle and add to the graduate to bring the final volume to 100 mL.

NOTES

GENERIC NAME	**Hydrocortisone**
DOSAGE FORM	oral suspension
MADE FROM	tablets
CONCENTRATION	2 mg/mL
STABILITY	14 days
STABILITY REFERENCE	Nahata MC, et al. Presented at: American Society of Health-System Pharmacists Midyear Meeting, December 2005 (poster)
STORE	refrigerate (preferable) or room temperature
LABEL	refrigerate, shake well before use

INGREDIENT	STRENGTH	QUANTITY
Hydrocortisone tablets	10 mg	20
Ora-Plus:Ora-Sweet	(1:1)	qs 100 mL

NOTE: The formulation in this study was stored in plastic amber bottles.

INSTRUCTIONS: Mix equal quantities of Ora-Plus and Ora-Sweet in a glass mortar by adding in geometric proportions to make 100 mL. Use this as the vehicle. Triturate the tablets into a fine powder in a glass mortar. Levigate the powder with a small portion of the vehicle into a smooth suspension. Add vehicle in geometric proportions, with constant mixing. Transfer the suspension to a graduate. Rinse the mortar with sufficient vehicle and add to the graduate to bring the final volume to 100 mL.

NOTES

GENERIC NAME	# Hydrocortisone
DOSAGE FORM	oral suspension
MADE FROM	tablets
CONCENTRATION	2 mg/mL
STABILITY	14 days
STABILITY REFERENCE	Nahata MC, et al. Presented at: American Society of Health-System Pharmacists Midyear Meeting, December 2005 (poster)
STORE	refrigerate (preferable) or room temperature
LABEL	refrigerate, shake well before use

INGREDIENT	STRENGTH	QUANTITY
Hydrocortisone tablets	10 mg	20
Simple syrup NF:1% methylcellulose	(1:1)	qs 100 mL

NOTE:	The formulation in this study was stored in plastic amber bottles.
INSTRUCTIONS:	Mix equal quantities of simple syrup, NF, and 1% methylcellulose in a glass mortar by adding in geometric proportions to make 100 mL. Use this as the vehicle. Triturate the tablets into a fine powder in a glass mortar. Levigate the powder with a small portion of the vehicle into a smooth suspension. Add vehicle in geometric proportions with constant mixing. Transfer the suspension to a graduate. Rinse the mortar with sufficient vehicle and add to the graduate to bring the final volume to 100 mL.

NOTES

Hydrocortisone Sodium Phosphate

GENERIC NAME	
DOSAGE FORM	injection
MADE FROM	injection
CONCENTRATION	5 mg/mL
STABILITY	7 days
STABILITY REFERENCE	experience
STORE	refrigerate
LABEL	refrigerate

INGREDIENT	STRENGTH	QUANTITY
Hydrocortisone sodium phosphate	50 mg/mL	3 mL
Bacteriostatic water for injection (parabens)		27 mL

NOTE: Use for ≤5-mg doses.
INSTRUCTIONS: Mix in a 30-mL empty sterile vial.

NOTES

GENERIC NAME	**Hydrocortisone/Neomycin**
DOSAGE FORM	enema
MADE FROM	powder
CONCENTRATION	10 mg/mL (hydrocortisone) / 8.35 mg/mL (neomycin)
STABILITY	30 days
STABILITY REFERENCE	experience
STORE	room temperature
LABEL	shake well before use, for rectal use only

INGREDIENT	STRENGTH	QUANTITY
Hydrocortisone powder		10.0 g
Neomycin powder		8.35 g
Polysorbate 80		10 mL
Methylcellulose	1%	
NaCl 0.9%		aa qs 1000 mL

INSTRUCTIONS: Prepare 1 L of the mixture of polysorbate 80, NaCl 0.9%, and methylcellulose 1%. Wet the hydrocortisone powder with a small amount of the above mixture by using a glass mortar and pestle, and continue to add the mixture to make a suspension. Dissolve the neomycin in 100 mL of the mixture and add to the hydrocortisone mixture, then qs to volume in a graduate.

NOTES

GENERIC NAME	**Hydroquinone**
DOSAGE FORM	ointment
MADE FROM	powder
CONCENTRATION	5% w/w
STABILITY	90 days
STABILITY REFERENCE	Matsubayashi T, et al. Biol Pharm Bull 2002; 25:92-6
STORE	refrigerate
LABEL	refrigerate

INGREDIENT	STRENGTH	QUANTITY
Hydroquinone, USP		5 g
L (+) Ascorbic acid, USP		1.6 g
Sodium sulfite, USP		0.5 g
Glycerin, USP		10 mL
Hydrophilic ointment		qs 100 g

NOTE: No information on storage container available.

INSTRUCTIONS: Add the solid ingredients to a glass mortar in geometric proportions and triturate into a fine powder. Add glycerin in small quantities and levigate into a smooth suspension. Add this suspension to the hydrophilic ointment in geometric proportions and levigate into a smooth ointment.

NOTES

GENERIC NAME	**Hydroquinone**
DOSAGE FORM	ointment
MADE FROM	powder
CONCENTRATION	10% w/w
STABILITY	90 days
STABILITY REFERENCE	Matsubayashi T, et al. Biol Pharm Bull 2002; 25:92-6
STORE	refrigerate
LABEL	refrigerate

INGREDIENT	STRENGTH	QUANTITY
Hydroquinone, USP		10 g
L (+) Ascorbic acid, USP		1.6 g
Sodium sulfite, USP		0.5 g
Glycerin, USP		10 mL
Hydrophilic ointment		qs 100 g

NOTE: No information on storage container available.

INSTRUCTIONS: Add the solid ingredients to a glass mortar in geometric proportions and triturate into a fine powder. Add glycerin in small quantities and levigate into a smooth suspension. Add this suspension to the hydrophilic ointment in geometric proportions and levigate into a smooth ointment.

NOTES

GENERIC NAME	**Hydroxychloroquine**
DOSAGE FORM	oral suspension
MADE FROM	tablets
CONCENTRATION	25 mg/mL
STABILITY	30 days
STABILITY REFERENCE	Pesko LJ. Am Druggist 1993;207:57
STORE	refrigerate
LABEL	shake well before use, refrigerate

INGREDIENT	STRENGTH	QUANTITY
Hydroxychloroquine sulfate tablets, USP	200 mg	15
Ora-Plus		60 mL
Water for irrigation, USP		qs 120 mL

NOTE:	In this study, the formulation was stored in amber glass bottles. Stability-indicating analytical methods not used.
INSTRUCTIONS:	Remove the coating of the hydroxychloroquine tablets with a towel moistened with alcohol. Crush the tablets to a fine powder using a glass mortar and pestle. Add 15 mL of Ora-Plus to the powder and levigate to a fine paste. Add the remaining Ora-Plus to the paste in geometric proportions. Transfer the mixture to a graduate. Using small amounts of water, rinse the mortar, transfer to the graduate, and qs to 120 mL.

NOTES

GENERIC NAME	**Hydroxypropylmethylcellulose solution**
DOSAGE FORM	oral suspension
MADE FROM	powder
CONCENTRATION	1%
STABILITY	6 months
STABILITY REFERENCE	Helin-Tanninen M, et al. Clin Pharm Ther 2001;26:59-66
STORE	room temperature
LABEL	shake well before use

INGREDIENT	STRENGTH	QUANTITY
Hydroxypropylmethylcellulose, USP		1 g
Purified water, USP		qs 100 mL

INSTRUCTIONS: Heat ~30 mL of water to 80–90 °C in a glass beaker calibrated to 100 mL, and mix with hydroxypropylmethylcellulose with vigorous stirring until the agglomerates disappear and the particles are thoroughly wetted. Add cold water (~5 °C) to volume. Continue stirring gently until the mixture is homogenous. Cool the solution in icy water until thoroughly hydrated, then allow it to gradually warm to ambient temperature. Autoclave at 121 °C for 20 minutes. Allow to cool to room temperature.

NOTES

GENERIC NAME	**Hydroxyurea**
DOSAGE FORM	oral solution
MADE FROM	capsules
CONCENTRATION	100 mg/mL
STABILITY	90 days
STABILITY REFERENCE	Heeney MM, et al. J Pediatr Hematol Oncol 2004;26:179-84
STORE	room temperature
LABEL	do not refrigerate; may form crystals

INGREDIENT	STRENGTH	QUANTITY
Hydroxyurea capsules	500 mg	10
Sterile water		25 mL
Syrpalta (flavored, not colored)		qs 50 mL

NOTE: This formulation should be prepared in a biological safety cabinet with proper personnel protective equipment.

INSTRUCTIONS: Mix the contents of the capsules with 25 mL of sterile water in a glass beaker, with constant vigorous stirring for a few hours. Filter the solution into a graduate to remove all insoluble capsule excipients. Mix this solution in geometric proportions with small quantities of Syrpalta, with constant stirring, to bring the final volume to 50 mL.

NOTES

GENERIC NAME	**Hydroxyurea**
DOSAGE FORM	oral solution
MADE FROM	powder
CONCENTRATION	100 mg/mL
STABILITY	90 days
STABILITY REFERENCE	experience, Heeney MM, et al. J Pediatr Hematol Oncol 2004;26:179-84
STORE	room temperature
LABEL	do not refrigerate; may form crystals

INGREDIENT	STRENGTH	QUANTITY
Hydroxyurea powder		25 g
Sterile water irrigation		125 mL
Simple syrup, NF		qs 250 mL

NOTE: This formulation should be prepared in a biological safety cabinet with proper personnel protective equipment.

INSTRUCTIONS: Mix the powder with small increments of sterile water in a glass beaker, with constant vigorous stirring for a few hours until the powder is completely dissolved. Mix this solution in geometric proportions with small quantities of simple syrup, with constant stirring, to bring the final volume to 250 mL.

NOTES

GENERIC NAME	**Indomethacin**
DOSAGE FORM	oral suspension
MADE FROM	capsules
CONCENTRATION	2 mg/mL
STABILITY	30 days
STABILITY REFERENCE	Gupta VD, et al. Am J Hosp Pharm 1978;35: 1382-5
STORE	room temperature
LABEL	shake well before use

INGREDIENT	STRENGTH	QUANTITY
Indomethacin capsules	25 mg	4
Ethanol	95%	10 mL
Methylparabens	0.005%	
Propylparabens	0.002%	
Simple syrup, NF		qs 50 mL

NOTE: In this study, the formulation was stored in amber bottles. Stability-indicating analytical methods not used. Commercially available as an oral suspension, 25 mg/ 5 mL.

INSTRUCTIONS: Empty the contents of the capsules in a mortar and mix well. Wet with ethanol and levigate into a smooth paste. Add the parabens and mix well. Add simple syrup in geometric proportions, mix well, and transfer to a graduate. Rinse the mortar with simple syrup, transfer to a graduate, and qs to 50 mL.

NOTES

GENERIC NAME	**Isoniazid**
DOSAGE FORM	oral suspension
MADE FROM	tablets
CONCENTRATION	10 mg/mL
STABILITY	21 days
STABILITY REFERENCE	experience
STORE	refrigerate
LABEL	shake well before use, refrigerate

INGREDIENT	STRENGTH	QUANTITY
Isoniazid tablets	100 mg	10
Purified water, USP		10 mL
Sorbitol solution	70%	qs ad 100 mL

NOTE: Do not use sugar-based solutions. Commercially available as a syrup, 50 mg/5 mL.

INSTRUCTIONS: Triturate the tablets in a mortar with water. Transfer to a graduate and qs with sorbitol solution.

NOTES

GENERIC NAME	**Isoniazid**
DOSAGE FORM	oral suspension
MADE FROM	powder
CONCENTRATION	10 mg/mL
STABILITY	28 days
STABILITY REFERENCE	Seifart HI, et al. Pediatr Infect Dis J 1991;10: 827-31
STORE	refrigerate (preferable) or at room temperature
LABEL	shake well before use, refrigerate

INGREDIENT	STRENGTH	QUANTITY
Isoniazid powder		1500 mg
Sodium sulfate		1800 mg
Glycerin		30 mL
Aqua chloroform concentrate		3 mL
Coloring agent (apple green)		0.45 mL
Water		qs 150 mL

NOTE: Stability-indicating analytical methods not used. Commercially available as a syrup, 50 mg/5 mL.

INSTRUCTIONS: Dissolve isoniazid and sodium sulfate in approximately 15 mL of water. Mix with glycerin, chloroform, water, and coloring agent in geometric proportions in a graduate. Add water and qs to 150 mL.

NOTES

GENERIC NAME	**Isradipine**
DOSAGE FORM	oral suspension
MADE FROM	capsules
CONCENTRATION	1 mg/mL
STABILITY	35 days
STABILITY REFERENCE	McDonald JL, et al. Am J Hosp Pharm 1994;51: 2409-11
STORE	refrigerate
LABEL	shake well before use, refrigerate

INGREDIENT	STRENGTH	QUANTITY
Isradipine capsules	5 mg	10
Glycerin, USP		qs ad 50 mL
Simple syrup, NF		qs

NOTE: In this study, the formulation was stored in type III amber glass prescription bottles.

INSTRUCTIONS: Empty the contents of the capsules and triturate to a fine powder. Add glycerin, USP, to wet the powder and levigate to a fine paste. Add approximately 15 mL of simple syrup to the paste in geometric proportions and triturate well. Transfer to a graduate. Rinse the mortar with 10 mL of simple syrup and transfer the contents to the graduate. Repeat rinsing and qs to 50 mL.

NOTES

GENERIC NAME	**Itraconazole**
DOSAGE FORM	oral suspension
MADE FROM	capsules
CONCENTRATION	20 mg/mL
STABILITY	56 days
STABILITY REFERENCE	Abdel-Rahman S, et al. J Ped Pharm Pract 1998; 3:115-8
STORE	refrigerate (preferable) or at room temperature
LABEL	shake well before use, refrigerate

INGREDIENT	STRENGTH	QUANTITY
Itraconazole capsules	100 mg	40
Alcohol, USP		15 mL
Ora-Plus		
Ora-Sweet		aa qs 200 mL

NOTE: In this study, the formulation was stored in amber plastic prescription bottles. Commercially available as an oral solution, 100 mg/10 mL.

INSTRUCTIONS: Empty the contents of the capsules into a mortar and add the alcohol. Let stand for 5 minutes. Mix the Ora-Sweet and Ora-Plus together. Triturate the beads to a fine powder and add the mixture in small amounts while mixing.

NOTES

GENERIC NAME	**Itraconazole**
DOSAGE FORM	oral suspension
MADE FROM	capsules
CONCENTRATION	40 mg/mL
STABILITY	35 days (2–6 °C)
STABILITY REFERENCE	Jacobson PA, et al. Am J Health Syst Pharm 1995;52:189-91
STORE	refrigerate, in amber glass
LABEL	shake well before use, refrigerate, protect from light

INGREDIENT	STRENGTH	QUANTITY
Itraconazole capsules	100 mg	24
Ethyl alcohol, USP		5 mL
Simple Syrup, NF		qs ad 60 mL

NOTE: In this study, the formulation was stored in type III amber glass prescription bottles. Commercially available as an oral solution, 100 mg/10 mL.

INSTRUCTIONS: Empty the beads from the capsules into a glass mortar. Add alcohol to the beads and let stand 3–4 minutes to soften the beads. Triturate with a pestle until alcohol evaporates and a dry powder remains. Add syrup in small amounts while mixing. Transfer to a graduate and qs to 60 mL with syrup.

NOTES

GENERIC NAME	**Ketoconazole**
DOSAGE FORM	oral suspension
MADE FROM	tablets
CONCENTRATION	20 mg/mL
STABILITY	60 days
STABILITY REFERENCE	Allen LV Jr, et al. Am J Health Syst Pharm 1996; 53:2073-8
STORE	refrigerate (preferable) or at room temperature
LABEL	shake well before use, refrigerate

INGREDIENT	STRENGTH	QUANTITY
Ketoconazole tablets	200 mg	12
Ora-Plus:Ora-Sweet or Ora-Plus:Ora-Sweet SF		aa qs 120 mL

NOTE: In this study, the formulation was stored in amber clear plastic (polyethylene terephthalate) prescription ovals.

INSTRUCTIONS: Crush the tablets and triturate to a fine powder. Add approximately 20 mL of vehicle and levigate to a uniform paste. Add vehicle in geometric proportions almost to volume, mix thoroughly, and transfer to a graduate. Rinse the mortar with vehicle, add to the graduate, and qs to 120 mL.

NOTES

GENERIC NAME	**Ketoconazole**
DOSAGE FORM	oral suspension
MADE FROM	tablets
CONCENTRATION	20 mg/mL
STABILITY	60 days
STABILITY REFERENCE	Allen LV Jr, et al. Am J Health Syst Pharm 1996;53:2073-8
STORE	refrigerate (preferable) or at room temperature
LABEL	shake well before use, refrigerate

INGREDIENT	STRENGTH	QUANTITY
Ketoconazole tablets	200 mg	12
Cherry syrup (cherry syrup concentrate diluted 1:4 with simple syrup, NF)		qs 120 mL

NOTE: In this study, the formulation was stored in amber clear polyethylene terephthalate prescription ovals.

INSTRUCTIONS: Crush the tablets and triturate to a fine powder. Add approximately 20 mL of vehicle and levigate to a uniform paste. Add vehicle in geometric proportions almost to volume, mix thoroughly, and transfer to a graduate. Rinse the mortar with vehicle, add to the graduate, and qs to 120 mL.

NOTES

GENERIC NAME	**Labetalol**
DOSAGE FORM	oral suspension
MADE FROM	tablets
CONCENTRATION	10 mg/mL
STABILITY	28 days
STABILITY REFERENCE	Nahata MC. DICP 1991;25:465-9
STORE	refrigerate (preferable) or at room temperature
LABEL	shake well before use, refrigerate

INGREDIENT	STRENGTH	QUANTITY
Labetalol tablets	100 mg	10
Simple syrup, NF		qs ad 100 mL

NOTE: In this study, the formulation was stored in amber plastic and glass prescription ovals. Stability-indicating analytical methods not used.

INSTRUCTIONS: Triturate the tablets to a fine powder in a mortar. Add a small quantity of syrup and stir to make a paste. Add increasing amounts of syrup while mixing. Transfer to a graduate and qs to desired volume with syrup.

NOTES

GENERIC NAME	**Labetalol**
DOSAGE FORM	oral suspension
MADE FROM	tablets
CONCENTRATION	40 mg/mL
STABILITY	60 days
STABILITY REFERENCE	Allen LV Jr, et al. Am J Health Syst Pharm 1996;53:2304-8
STORE	refrigerate (preferable) or at room temperature
LABEL	shake well before use, refrigerate

INGREDIENT	STRENGTH	QUANTITY
Labetalol hydrochloride tablets	300 mg	16
Ora-Plus:Ora-Sweet	1:1	
or Ora-Plus:Ora-Sweet SF	1:1	qs 120 mL

NOTE: In this study, the formulation was stored in amber clear plastic (polyethylene terephthalate) prescription ovals.

INSTRUCTIONS: Crush the tablets and triturate to a fine powder. Add approximately 20 mL of vehicle and levigate to a uniform paste. Add vehicle in geometric proportions almost to volume, mix thoroughly, and transfer to a graduate. Rinse the mortar with vehicle, add to the graduate, and qs to 120 mL.

NOTES

GENERIC NAME	**Labetalol**
DOSAGE FORM	oral suspension
MADE FROM	tablets
CONCENTRATION	40 mg/mL
STABILITY	60 days
STABILITY REFERENCE	Allen LV Jr, et al. Am J Health Syst Pharm 1996; 53:2304-8
STORE	refrigerate (preferable) or at room temperature
LABEL	shake well before use, refrigerate

INGREDIENT	STRENGTH	QUANTITY
Labetalol tablets	300 mg	16
Cherry syrup concentrate (diluted 1:4 with simple syrup, NF)		qs 120 mL

NOTE: In this study, the formulation was stored in amber clear plastic (polyethylene terephthalate) prescription ovals.

INSTRUCTIONS: Crush the tablets and triturate to a fine powder. Add approximately 20 mL of vehicle and levigate to a uniform paste. Add vehicle in geometric proportions almost to volume, mix thoroughly, and transfer to a graduate. Rinse the mortar with vehicle, add to the graduate, and qs to 120 mL.

NOTES

GENERIC NAME	**Lamotrigine**
DOSAGE FORM	oral suspension
MADE FROM	tablets
CONCENTRATION	1 mg/mL
STABILITY	91 days
STABILITY REFERENCE	Nahata MC, et al. Am J Health Syst Pharm 1999;56:240-2
STORE	refrigerate (preferable) or at room temperature
LABEL	shake well before use, refrigerate

INGREDIENT	STRENGTH	QUANTITY
Lamotrigine tablet	100 mg	1
Ora-Plus:Ora-Sweet or Ora-Plus:Ora-Sweet SF	1:1	qs 100 mL

NOTE: In this study, the formulation was stored in amber clear plastic (polyethylene terephthalate) prescription bottles.

INSTRUCTIONS: Crush the tablets in a mortar and triturate to a fine powder. Add a small amount of vehicle and mix to a uniform paste. Add geometric proportions of the vehicle while mixing to almost 100 mL. Transfer the mixture to a graduate and qs to 100 mL with vehicle. Mix well.

NOTES

GENERIC NAME	**Lansoprazole**
DOSAGE FORM	oral suspension
MADE FROM	capsules
CONCENTRATION	3 mg/mL
STABILITY	14 days
STABILITY REFERENCE	DiGiacinto JL, et al. Ann Pharmacother 2000;34: 600-5
STORE	refrigerate
LABEL	shake well before use, refrigerate

INGREDIENT	STRENGTH	QUANTITY
Lansoprazole capsules	30 mg	10
Sodium bicarbonate injection, USP	8.4%	100 mL

NOTE: In this study, the formulation was stored in amber plastic oral syringes.

INSTRUCTIONS: Empty contents of capsules into a 250-mL Erlenmeyer flask. Measure 100 mL of sodium bicarbonate solution in a graduate and add to the flask. Stir the mixture with a magnetic stirrer for 30 minutes.

NOTES

GENERIC NAME	**Levodopa/Carbidopa**
DOSAGE FORM	oral suspension
MADE FROM	tablets
CONCENTRATION	5 mg/mL (levodopa) and 1.25 mg/mL (carbidopa)
STABILITY	42 days (4 °C); 14 days (25 °C)
STABILITY REFERENCE	Nahata MC, et al. J Pediatr Ophthalmol Strabismus 2000;37:333-7
STORE	refrigerate
LABEL	shake well before use, refrigerate

INGREDIENT	STRENGTH	QUANTITY
Sinemet tablets	100 mg/25 mg	10
Ora-Sweet		100 mL
Ora-Plus		100 mL

NOTE: In this study, the formulation was stored in amber plastic prescription bottles.

INSTRUCTIONS: Crush tablets in a mortar and reduce to a fine powder. Add a small amount of the vehicle to the powder and mix to a uniform paste. Add geometric amounts of the mixture almost to volume while mixing. Transfer to a graduate and qs with vehicle to volume.

NOTES

GENERIC NAME	**Levofloxacin**
DOSAGE FORM	oral suspension
MADE FROM	tablets
CONCENTRATION	50 mg/mL
STABILITY	57 days
STABILITY REFERENCE	VandenBussche HL, et al. Am J Health Syst Pharm 1999;56:2316-8
STORE	refrigerate (preferable) or at room temperature
LABEL	shake well before use, refrigerate

INGREDIENT	STRENGTH	QUANTITY
Levofloxacin tablets	500 mg	6
Ora-Plus/strawberry syrup, NF		aa qs 60 mL

NOTE: In this study, the formulation was stored in amber plastic prescription bottles.

INSTRUCTIONS: Crush the tablets in a mortar and reduce to a fine powder. Add a small amount of the vehicle to the mortar and mix to a uniform paste. Add additional vehicle almost to volume while mixing. Transfer to a graduate and qs to volume of 60 mL.

NOTES

GENERIC NAME	**Levothyroxine**
DOSAGE FORM	oral suspension
MADE FROM	tablets
CONCENTRATION	25 mcg/mL
STABILITY	8 days
STABILITY REFERENCE	Boulton DV, et al. Am J Health Syst Pharm 1996;53:1157-61
STORE	refrigerate
LABEL	shake well before use, refrigerate

INGREDIENT	STRENGTH	QUANTITY
Levothyroxine sodium tablets	0.1 mg	25
Glycerin		40 mL
Water		qs 100 mL

NOTE: In this study, the formulation was stored in amber high-density polyethylene bottles.

INSTRUCTIONS: Triturate the tablets in a mortar to fine powder. Levigate the powder with small amounts of glycerin into a smooth paste. Add more glycerin in geometric proportions until the suspension is pourable. Transfer the suspension into a 100-mL graduate. Rinse the mortar with water repeatedly, transfer to the graduate, and qs to 100 mL.

NOTES

GENERIC NAME	**Levothyroxine**
DOSAGE FORM	oral suspension
MADE FROM	tablets
CONCENTRATION	25 mcg/mL
STABILITY	14 days refrigerated; 7 days room temperature
STABILITY REFERENCE	Nahata MC, et al. Presented at: American Society of Health-System Pharmacists Midyear Clinical Meeting, December 2005 (poster)
STORE	refrigerate (preferable) or room temperature
LABEL	refrigerate, shake well before use

INGREDIENT	STRENGTH	QUANTITY
Levothyroxine tablets	200 mcg	10
Simple syrup, NF: 1% methylcellulose suspension	1:10	qs 80 mL

NOTE: This formulation was stored in amber prescription bottles.

INSTRUCTIONS: Mix simple syrup and 1% methylcellulose suspension thoroughly together in a glass mortar, in geometric proportions, to prepare the vehicle. Triturate the tablets into a fine powder and levigate with small proportion of the vehicle into a smooth suspension. Add vehicle in geometric proportions with constant mixing. Transfer to a graduate. Rinse the mortar with sufficient vehicle and transfer to graduate to make up the final volume.

NOTES

GENERIC NAME	**Levothyroxine**
DOSAGE FORM	oral suspension
MADE FROM	tablets
CONCENTRATION	25 mcg/mL
STABILITY	14 days refrigerated; 7 days room temperature
STABILITY REFERENCE	Nahata MC, et al. Presented at: American Society of Health-System Pharmacists Midyear Clinical Meeting, December 2005
STORE	refrigerate or room temperature
LABEL	refrigerate, shake well before use

INGREDIENT	STRENGTH	QUANTITY
Levothyroxine tablets	200 mcg	10
Ora-Plus:Ora-Sweet	1:1	qs 80 mL

NOTE: This formulation was stored in amber prescription bottles.

INSTRUCTIONS: Mix Ora-Plus and Ora-Sweet together thoroughly in a glass mortar pestle, in geometric proportions, to prepare the vehicle. Triturate the tablets into a fine powder and levigate with small proportion of the vehicle into a smooth suspension. Add vehicle in geometric proportions, with constant mixing. Transfer to a graduate. Rinse the mortar and pestle with sufficient vehicle and transfer to graduate to make up the final volume.

NOTES

Lidocaine, Epinephrine, and Tetracaine (LET) Solution

GENERIC NAME	
DOSAGE FORM	topical anesthetic solution
CONCENTRATION	lidocaine hydrochloride 40 mg/mL, racepinephrine 2.25 mg/mL, tetracaine hydrochloride 5 mg/mL
STABILITY	182 days (4 °C); 28 days (18 °C)
STABILITY REFERENCE	Larson TA, et al. Am J Health Syst Pharm 1996; 53:659-62
STORE	refrigerate
LABEL	refrigerate, for topical use only

INGREDIENT	STRENGTH	QUANTITY
Lidocaine hydrochloride injection	20%	10 mL
Racepinephrine (as hydrochloride salt)	2.25%	5 mL
Tetracaine hydrochloride	2%	12.5 mL
Sodium metabisulfite		0.0315 g
Sterile water for irrigation		22.5 mL

NOTE: The solution should have a blue tint in a clear container. In this study, the formulation was stored in amber glass containers. Stability-indicating analytical methods used only for epinephrine.

INSTRUCTIONS: Measure 10 mL of lidocaine hydrochloride injection 20%, 5 mL of racepinephrine 2.25%, 12.5 mL of tetracaine hydrochloride 2%, and 22.5 mL of sterile water for irrigation. Weigh out 0.0315 g of sodium metabisulfite. Transfer all the ingredients to an amber glass container with a tight-fitting cap. Mix well.

NOTES

Lidocaine, Epinephrine, and Tetracaine (LET II) Gel

GENERIC NAME	
DOSAGE FORM	topical anesthetic gel
MADE FROM	
CONCENTRATION	lidocaine 4%, epinephrine 0.05%, tetracaine 0.5%
STABILITY	150 days refrigerated
STABILITY REFERENCE	21 days room temperature
STORE	experience
LABEL	refrigerate (preferred) or room temperature, refrigerate, protect from light

INGREDIENT	STRENGTH	QUANTITY
Epinephrine bitartrate, USP		0.32 g
Lidocaine hydrochloride, USP		8 g
Lidocaine jelly 2% (30 mL tube)		300 mL
Sodium bisulfate		0.26 g
Sterile water for injection		50 mL
Tetracaine USP (free base)		1.75 g

NOTE: This formulation should be prepared in a laminar air flow hood and stored in amber, plastic 5-mL oral syringes.

INSTRUCTIONS: Glass beaker, glass mortar and pestle, and glass stirrer used for this formulation are cleaned with hot water, rinsed with sterile water for irrigation, and thoroughly dried. Before use, clean with isopropyl alcohol 70%. Alternatively, these utensils can be sterilized using other methods available. In a laminar flow hood, mix tetracaine, sodium bisulfate, lidocaine HCl, and epinephrine bitartrate powders in a beaker in geometric proportions, add sterile water for injection, and stir to dissolve. Draw this solution into a 60-mL sterile syringe and attach a 0.2-μ filter. In a glass mortar, add lidocaine jelly and stir using a glass rod. Inject the solution through the filter into the mortar, adding geometrically, and stir with the glass rod in a figure of 8 to avoid introducing air bubbles. Allow to sit in laminar air flow hood to allow air bubbles to dissipate. Draw dose of 3 mL into amber plastic 5-mL oral syringes by placing the tip of the syringe in the gel. Clean the tip with alcohol and place the cap. Seal the cap with a tamper-resistant seal.

NOTES

GENERIC NAME	**Lisinopril**
DOSAGE FORM	oral suspension
MADE FROM	tablets
CONCENTRATION	1 mg/mL
STABILITY	90 days
STABILITY REFERENCE	Nahata MC, et al. Presented at: American Society of Health-System Pharmacists Midyear Clinical Meeting, New Orleans, December 2–6, 2001 (poster)
STORE	refrigerate (preferable) or at room temperature
LABEL	shake well before use, refrigerate

INGREDIENT	STRENGTH	QUANTITY
Lisinopril tablets	10 mg	10
Ora-Plus		
Ora-Sweet		aa qs 100 mL

NOTE: In this study, the formulation was stored in plastic prescription bottles.

INSTRUCTIONS: Crush the tablets and triturate to a fine powder in a mortar. Levigate the powder with a small amount of the vehicle into a uniform paste. Add the vehicle in geometric proportions with constant mixing and transfer to a graduate. Rinse the mortar with vehicle, transfer to the graduate, and qs to 100 mL.

NOTES

GENERIC NAME	**Lisinopril**
DOSAGE FORM	oral suspension
MADE FROM	tablets
CONCENTRATION	1 mg/mL
STABILITY	90 days (4 °C); 56 days (25 °C)
STABILITY REFERENCE	Nahata MC, et al. Presented at: American Society of Health-System Pharmacists Midyear Clinical Meeting, New Orleans, December 2–6, 2001 (poster)
STORE	refrigerate (preferable) or at room temperature
LABEL	shake well before use, refrigerate

INGREDIENT	STRENGTH	QUANTITY
Lisinopril tablets	10 mg	10
Methylcellulose	1% with parabens	7 mL
Simple syrup, NF		qs 100 mL

NOTE: In this study, the formulation was stored in plastic prescription bottles.

INSTRUCTIONS: Crush the tablets and triturate to a fine powder in a mortar. Levigate the powder with methylcellulose gel into a uniform paste. Add simple syrup in geometric proportions with constant mixing and transfer to a graduate. Rinse the mortar with syrup and transfer to the graduate and qs to 100 mL.

NOTES

Copyright © 2011 Harvey Whitney Books

GENERIC NAME	**Lisinopril**
DOSAGE FORM	oral suspension
MADE FROM	tablets
CONCENTRATION	1 mg/mL
STABILITY	28 days
STABILITY REFERENCE	Thompson KC, et al. Am J Health Syst Pharm 2003;60:69-74
STORE	room temperature
LABEL	shake well before use

INGREDIENT	STRENGTH	QUANTITY
Lisinopril	20 mg	10
Purified water		10 mL
Bicitra		30 mL
Ora-Sweet SF		160 mL

NOTE: In this study, the formulation was stored in amber polyethylene terephthalate containers with screw caps. Bicitra contains sodium citrate dihydrate (500 mg/5 mL) and citric acid monohydrate (334 mg/5 mL).

INSTRUCTIONS: Place 10 tablets and 10 mL of purified water into an 8-oz amber polyethylene terephthalate container. Place the screw cap on and shake the solution for at least 1 minute. Add 30 mL of Bicitra solution and shake the bottle again, ensuring that the tablets have disintegrated into a uniform suspension. Add 160 mL of Ora-Sweet SF solution and disperse the contents to make a uniform suspension.

NOTES

GENERIC NAME	**Lorazepam**
DOSAGE FORM	oral suspension
MADE FROM	tablets
CONCENTRATION	1 mg/mL
STABILITY	63 days
STABILITY REFERENCE	Wan-Man EL, et al. Int J Pharmaceut Compd 2004;9:254-8
STORE	refrigerate (preferable) or room temperature
LABEL	refrigerate, shake well before use

INGREDIENT	STRENGTH	QUANTITY
Lorazepam tablets	1 mg	120
Distilled water		20 mL
Ora-Plus:Ora-Sweet	1:1	qs 120 mL

NOTE: No information on storage containers provided.

INSTRUCTIONS: Mix Ora-Plus and Ora-Sweet together thoroughly in a glass mortar pestle, in geometric proportions, to prepare the vehicle. Triturate the tablets into a fine powder and levigate with small proportion of distilled water into a smooth suspension. Add vehicle in geometric proportions, with constant mixing. Transfer to a graduate. Rinse the mortar and pestle with sufficient vehicle and transfer to graduate to make up the final volume.

NOTES

GENERIC NAME	**Lorazepam, Diluted**
DOSAGE FORM	injection
MADE FROM	injection
CONCENTRATION	1 mg/mL
STABILITY	7 days
STABILITY REFERENCE	Nahata MC, et al. Presented at: American Society of Health-System Pharmacists Midyear Clinical Meeting, New Orleans, December 2–6, 2001 (poster)
STORE	refrigerate, in an empty sterile glass vial
LABEL	refrigerate

INGREDIENT	STRENGTH	QUANTITY
Lorazepam injection	4 mg/mL	1 mL
Bacteriostatic water for injection		3 mL

INSTRUCTIONS: Mix the two ingredients aseptically in a syringe in a laminar flow hood.

NOTES

GENERIC NAME	**Losartan**
DOSAGE FORM	oral suspension
MADE FROM	tablets
CONCENTRATION	2.5 mg/mL
STABILITY	28 days
STABILITY REFERENCE	Cozaar package insert, www.merck.com/product/usa/picirculars/c/cozaar/cozaar_pi.pdf (accessed 2010 Jul 24)
STORE	refrigerate
LABEL	refrigerate, shake well before use

INGREDIENT	STRENGTH	QUANTITY
Losartan tablets	50 mg	10
Distilled water		10 mL
Ora-Plus:Ora-Sweet SF	1:1	qs 200 mL

NOTE: The formulation was stored in amber prescription bottles.
INSTRUCTIONS: Place the tablets in an amber plastic prescription bottle and add distilled water. Cap and shake mixture for 2 minutes. Allow to stand for 1 hour and then shake for 1 minute. Add vehicle to bottle and shake for 1 minute.

NOTES

GENERIC NAME	**Mercaptopurine**
DOSAGE FORM	oral suspension
MADE FROM	tablets
CONCENTRATION	5 mg/mL
STABILITY	90 days
STABILITY REFERENCE	Nahata MC, et al. Presented at: American Society of Health-System Pharmacists Midyear Clinical Meeting, New Orleans, December 2–6, 2001 (poster)
STORE	refrigerate (preferable) or at room temperature
LABEL	shake well before use, refrigerate

INGREDIENT	STRENGTH	QUANTITY
Mercaptopurine tablets	50 mg	10
Ora-Plus		
Ora-Sweet		aa qs 100 mL

NOTE: In this study, the formulation was stored in plastic prescription bottles.

INSTRUCTIONS: Triturate the tablets in a glass mortar to a fine powder. Levigate the powder with small amounts of the vehicle into a uniform paste. Add vehicle in geometric proportions and transfer the suspension to a graduate. Rinse the mortar with the vehicle, add to the graduate, and qs to 100 mL.

NOTES

GENERIC NAME	**Mercaptopurine**
DOSAGE FORM	oral suspension
MADE FROM	tablets
CONCENTRATION	5 mg/mL
STABILITY	90 days (4 °C); 56 days (25 °C)
STABILITY REFERENCE	Nahata MC, et al. Presented at: American Society of Health-System Pharmacists Midyear Clinical Meeting, New Orleans, December 2–6, 2001 (poster)
STORE	refrigerate (preferable) or at room temperature
LABEL	shake well before use, refrigerate

INGREDIENT	STRENGTH	QUANTITY
Mercaptopurine tablets	50 mg	10
Methylcellulose	1% with parabens	10 mL
Simple syrup, NF		qs 100 mL

NOTE: In this study, the formulation was stored in plastic prescription bottles.

INSTRUCTIONS: Crush the tablets and triturate to a fine powder in a mortar. Levigate the powder with methylcellulose gel into a uniform paste. Add simple syrup in geometric proportions with constant mixing and transfer to a graduate. Rinse the mortar with syrup, transfer to the graduate, and qs to 100 mL.

NOTES

GENERIC NAME	# Mercaptopurine
DOSAGE FORM	oral suspension
MADE FROM	tablets
CONCENTRATION	50 mg/mL
STABILITY	14 days
STABILITY REFERENCE	Dressman JB, et al. Am J Hosp Pharm 1983;40: 616-8
STORE	room temperature
LABEL	shake well before use

INGREDIENT	STRENGTH	QUANTITY
Mercaptopurine tablets	50 mg	100
Methylcellulose solution	1%	
Simple syrup, NF		aa qs 100 mL

NOTE: Stability-indicating analytical methods not used. In this study, the formulation contained Cologel 33 mL and wild cherry syrup:simple syrup, NF (1:2) qs 100 mL of 50 mg/mL of the formulation. Cologel, a commercially available vehicle consisting of methylcellulose 9% solution, is no longer available. In the above formulation, Cologel can be substituted with methylcellulose solution 1% and the wild cherry syrup:simple syrup mixture with simple syrup, NF.

INSTRUCTIONS: Crush the tablets and triturate to a fine powder. Make a mixture of equal parts of syrup and methylcellulose. Add a small amount of this vehicle and levigate to a uniform paste. Add vehicle in geometric proportions almost to volume, mix thoroughly, and transfer to a graduate. Rinse the mortar with vehicle, add to the graduate, and qs to 100 mL.

NOTES

GENERIC NAME	**MESNA**
DOSAGE FORM	oral solution
MADE FROM	injection
CONCENTRATION	16.67 mg/mL, 33.33 mg/mL
STABILITY	7 days
STABILITY REFERENCE	Goren MP, et al. Cancer Chemother Pharmacol 1991;28:298-301
STORE	room temperature

INGREDIENT	STRENGTH	QUANTITY
MESNA injection	100 mg/mL vials	qs to administer the dose
Orange-flavored syrup or grape-flavored syrup		qs to 16.67 mg/mL or 33.33 mg/mL concentration

NOTE: In this study, the formulation was stored in capped glass tubes. Stability-indicating analytical methods not used.

INSTRUCTIONS: Mix MESNA with the appropriate amount of orange-flavored or grape-flavored syrup to obtain the desired concentration.

NOTES

GENERIC NAME	**MESNA**
DOSAGE FORM	oral solution
MADE FROM	injection
CONCENTRATION	1 mg/mL, 10 mg/mL, 50 mg/mL
STABILITY	7 days
STABILITY REFERENCE	Goren MP, et al. Cancer Chemother Pharmacol 1991;28:298-301
STORE	refrigerate
LABEL	refrigerate

INGREDIENT	STRENGTH	QUANTITY
MESNA injection	100 mg/mL vials	qs to administer the dose
Coca Cola or Dr. Pepper, or Sprite or 7-Up, or Pepsi Cola, or apple juice, or orange juice, or ginger ale		qs to obtain 50 mg/mL or 10 mg/mL or 1 mg/mL concentration

NOTE: In this study, the formulation was stored in capped glass tubes. Stability-indicating analytical methods not used.

INSTRUCTIONS: Mix MESNA with the appropriate amount of the chosen beverage to obtain the desired concentration.

NOTES

GENERIC NAME	**Methotrexate**
DOSAGE FORM	oral suspension
MADE FROM	powder
CONCENTRATION	0.5 mg/mL
STABILITY	14 days
STABILITY REFERENCE	Methotrexate 2.5 mg/5 mL oral liquid. Int J Pharmaceut Compd 1999;3:474
STORE	refrigerate, in amber-colored bottles
LABEL	shake well before use, refrigerate

INGREDIENT	STRENGTH	QUANTITY
Methotrexate powder		50 mg
Glycerin		2 mL
Ora-Plus		49 mL
Ora-Sweet or Ora-Sweet SF		49 mL

NOTE:	Stability-indicating analytical studies not used. Based on *United States Pharmacopeia XXIII/National Formulary 18* (Rockville, MD: US Pharmacopeial Convention, 1995:3531-5) beyond-use date recommendation for water-containing formulations in the absence of stability information.
INSTRUCTIONS:	Levigate the methotrexate powder to a paste with glycerin in a glass mortar. Add Ora-Plus in geometric proportions to this paste and form a suspension. Transfer the suspension to a 100-mL graduate. Rinse the mortar with small portions of Ora-Sweet or Ora-Sweet SF and add to the graduate.

NOTES

GENERIC NAME	**Methylcellulose**
DOSAGE FORM	oral suspension
MADE FROM	powder
CONCENTRATION	1%
STABILITY	6 months
STABILITY REFERENCE	experience
STORE	shake well before use, room temperature

INGREDIENT	STRENGTH	QUANTITY
Methylcellulose powder	4000 cps	10 g
Methylparaben		200 mg
Propylparaben		100 mg
Purified water, USP		qs 1000 mL

INSTRUCTIONS: Heat 200 mL of purified water to boiling. Add the parabens and mix well. Wet the methylcellulose powder and add it. Allow to stand for 15 minutes, then remove from heat. Then qs with cold purified water while mixing well with a magnetic stirrer. Keep mixing until a clear, homogenous solution results.

NOTES

GENERIC NAME	**Methyldopa**
DOSAGE FORM	oral suspension
MADE FROM	tablets
CONCENTRATION	50 mg/mL
STABILITY	14 days
STABILITY REFERENCE	Newton DW, et al. Am J Hosp Pharm 1975;32: 817-21
STORE	refrigerate (preferable) or at room temperature
LABEL	shake well before use, refrigerate

INGREDIENT	STRENGTH	QUANTITY
Methyldopa tablets	250 mg	2
Simple syrup, NF containing citric acid (0.5% w/v)		qs 10 mL

NOTE: Stability-indicating analytical methods not used. Commercially available as an oral suspension, 250 mg/mL.

INSTRUCTIONS: Crush the tablets in a mortar. Add syrups in small quantities while mixing. Adjust pH to 1.8 with 0.2N hydrochloric acid.

NOTES

GENERIC NAME	**Methyldopa**
DOSAGE FORM	oral suspension
MADE FROM	tablets
CONCENTRATION	50 mg/mL
STABILITY	14 days
STABILITY REFERENCE	Newton DW, et al. Am J Hosp Pharm 1975;32: 817-21
STORE	refrigerate (preferable) or at room temperature
LABEL	shake well before use, refrigerate

INGREDIENT	STRENGTH	QUANTITY
Methyldopa tablets	250 mg	10
Simple syrup, NF		qs 50 mL

NOTE: In this study, the formulation was stored in amber glass bottles. Stability-indicating analytical methods not used. Commercially available as an oral suspension, 250 mg/5 mL.

INSTRUCTIONS: Crush the tablets and triturate to a fine powder. Add approximately 20 mL of vehicle and levigate to a uniform paste. Add vehicle in geometric proportions almost to volume, mix thoroughly, and transfer to a graduate. Rinse the mortar with vehicle, add to the graduate, and qs to 50 mL.

NOTES

GENERIC NAME	**Methyldopa**
DOSAGE FORM	oral suspension
MADE FROM	tablets
CONCENTRATION	50 mg/mL
STABILITY	14 days
STABILITY REFERENCE	Newton DW, et al. Am J Hosp Pharm 1975;32: 817-21
STORE	refrigerate (preferable) or at room temperature
LABEL	shake well before use, refrigerate

INGREDIENT	STRENGTH	QUANTITY
Methyldopa tablets	250 mg	10
Hydrochloric acid	0.73% w/v, 0.2N	25 mL
Simple syrup, NF, containing 0.5% w/v citric acid		qs 50 mL

NOTE: The final solution should have a pH of 1.8. In this study, the formulation was stored in amber glass bottles. Stability-indicating analytical methods not used. Commercially available as an oral suspension, 250 mg/5 mL.

INSTRUCTIONS: Crush the tablets and triturate to a fine powder. Add 25 mL of the hydrochloric acid and levigate to a uniform paste. Add the citric acid syrup in geometric proportions almost to volume, mix thoroughly, and transfer to a graduate. Rinse the mortar with the citric acid syrup, add to the graduate, and qs to 50 mL.

NOTES

GENERIC NAME	**Methyldopa**
DOSAGE FORM	oral solution
MADE FROM	injection
CONCENTRATION	25 mg/mL
STABILITY	168 days
STABILITY REFERENCE	Gupta VD, et al. Am J Hosp Pharm 1978;35: 1382-5
STORE	room temperature

INGREDIENT	STRENGTH	QUANTITY
Methyldopa hydrochloride injection	50 mg/mL	5 vials (10 mL)
Sodium benzoate		0.1 g
Simple syrup, NF		qs 100 mL

NOTE: In this study, the formulation was stored in amber-colored bottles. Stability-indicating analytical methods not used. Commercially available as an oral suspension, 250 mg/5 mL.

INSTRUCTIONS: Dissolve sodium benzoate in approximately 5 mL of syrup mix with the methyldopa injection solution in geometric proportions and qs to 100 mL with simple syrup.

NOTES

GENERIC NAME	**Methyldopa**
DOSAGE FORM	oral solution
MADE FROM	powder
CONCENTRATION	25 mg/mL
STABILITY	168 days
STABILITY REFERENCE	Gupta VD, et al. Am J Hosp Pharm 1978;35: 1382-5
STORE	room temperature

INGREDIENT	STRENGTH	QUANTITY
Methyldopa hydrochloride powder		2.5 g
Sodium metabisulfite		0.1 g
Sodium edetate		0.1 g
Simple syrup, NF		qs 100 mL

NOTE: In this study, the formulation was stored in amber-colored bottles. Stability-indicating analytical methods not used. Commercially available as an oral suspension, 250 mg/5 mL.

INSTRUCTIONS: Dissolve methyldopa hydrochloride powder, sodium metabisulfite, and sodium edetate in approximately 20 mL of syrup, mix well, and qs to 100 mL with simple syrup.

NOTES

GENERIC NAME	**Methylphenidate**
DOSAGE FORM	oral suspension
MADE FROM	tablets
CONCENTRATION	any required concentration
STABILITY	15 days
STABILITY REFERENCE	Woods DJ. www.pharminfotech.co.nz/emixt
STORE	room temperature
LABEL	shake well before use

INGREDIENT	STRENGTH	QUANTITY
Methylphenidate hydrochloride tablets (Ritalin)		qs to obtain required concentration
Citric acid monohydrate		0.48 g
[a]Sodium citrate		0.072 g
[b]Parabens		0.1 %
Glycerin		50 mL
Water		qs 100 mL

[a]Can be omitted if not available. Addition of citric acid alone (qs to pH 3–4) is sufficient for short-term stability.
[b]Methyl hydroxybenzoate 4 g, propyl hydroxybenzoate 1 g, propylene glycol qs 100 mL. Mix 2 mL of this solution to 100 mL of formulation to give parabens 0.1%.

NOTE:	Stability-indicating analytical methods not used.
INSTRUCTIONS:	Crush the tablets and triturate to a fine powder. Levigate the powder with a sufficient amount of glycerin to form a uniform paste. Add the rest of the glycerin in geometric proportions and mix well. Dissolve citric acid and sodium citrate in approximately 5 mL of water. Add the parabens solution and the citric acid solution to the mortar in geometric proportions and mix well. Transfer to a graduate. Rinse the mortar with water, add to the graduate, and qs to 100 mL. Mix well.

NOTES

GENERIC NAME	**Methylprednisolone Sodium Succinate**
DOSAGE FORM	injection
MADE FROM	injection
CONCENTRATION	4 mg/mL
STABILITY	7 days
STABILITY REFERENCE	Nahata MC, et al. Am J Hosp Pharm 1994;51: 2157-9
STORE	refrigerate, store in an empty sterile vial
LABEL	refrigerate

INGREDIENT	STRENGTH	QUANTITY
Methylprednisolone injection	40 mg/mL	1 mL
Bacteriostatic water for injection, USP		9 mL

NOTE: In this study, the formulation was stored in glass vials.
INSTRUCTIONS: Mix the ingredients in a sterile syringe.

NOTES

GENERIC NAME	**Metolazone**
DOSAGE FORM	oral suspension
MADE FROM	tablets
CONCENTRATION	1 mg/mL
STABILITY	60 days
STABILITY REFERENCE	Allen LV Jr, et al. Am J Health Syst Pharm 1996; 53:2073-8
STORE	refrigerate (preferable) or at room temperature
LABEL	shake well before use, refrigerate

INGREDIENT	STRENGTH	QUANTITY
Metolazone tablets	10 mg	12
Ora-Plus:Ora-Sweet or Ora-Plus:Ora-Sweet SF	1:1	aa qs 120 mL

NOTE: In this study, the formulation was stored in amber clear plastic (polyethylene terephthalate) prescription ovals.

INSTRUCTIONS: Crush the tablets and triturate to a fine powder. Add approximately 20 mL of vehicle and levigate to a uniform paste. Add vehicle in geometric proportions almost to volume, mix thoroughly, and transfer to a graduate. Rinse the mortar with vehicle, add to the graduate, and qs to 120 mL.

NOTES

GENERIC NAME	**Metolazone**
DOSAGE FORM	oral suspension
MADE FROM	tablets
CONCENTRATION	1 mg/mL
STABILITY	60 days
STABILITY REFERENCE	Allen LV Jr, et al. Am J Health Syst Pharm 1996; 53:2073-8
STORE	refrigerate (preferable) or at room temperature
LABEL	shake well before use, refrigerate

INGREDIENT	STRENGTH	QUANTITY
Metolazone tablets	10 mg	12
Cherry syrup (cherry syrup concentrate diluted 1:4 with simple syrup, NF)		qs 120 mL

NOTE: In this study, the formulation was stored in amber clear plastic (polyethylene terephthalate) prescription ovals.

INSTRUCTIONS: Crush the tablets and triturate to a fine powder. Add approximately 20 mL of vehicle and levigate to a uniform paste. Add vehicle in geometric proportions almost to volume, mix thoroughly, and transfer to a graduate. Rinse the mortar with vehicle, add to the graduate, and qs to 120 mL.

NOTES

GENERIC NAME	**Metolazone**
DOSAGE FORM	oral suspension
MADE FROM	tablets
CONCENTRATION	0.25 mg/mL
STABILITY	91 days (4 °C glass and plastic); 28 days (25 °C plastic); 14 days (25 °C glass)
STABILITY REFERENCE	Nahata MC, et al. Hosp Pharm 1997;32:691-3
STORE	refrigerate
LABEL	shake well before use, refrigerate

INGREDIENT	STRENGTH	QUANTITY
Metolazone tablets	2.5 mg	10
Methylcellulose 1%	1:1	qs ad 100 mL
Simple syrup, NF		

NOTE: In this study, the formulation was stored in glass and plastic prescription bottles.

INSTRUCTIONS: Crush tablets in a glass mortar and triturate into a fine powder. Mix methylcellulose 1% suspension and simple syrup in geometric proportions to make the vehicle. Add small amount of vehicle and levigate the powder into a smooth suspension. Add more vehicle in geometric proportions with constant mixing. Transfer the suspension to a graduate, rinse the mortar with the vehicle, and add to graduate, with mixing to make up the final volume.

NOTES

GENERIC NAME	**Metoprolol**
DOSAGE FORM	oral suspension
MADE FROM	tablets
CONCENTRATION	10 mg/mL
STABILITY	60 days
STABILITY REFERENCE	Allen LV Jr, et al. Am J Health Syst Pharm 1996; 53:2304-8
STORE	refrigerate (preferable) or at room temperature
LABEL	shake well before use, refrigerate

INGREDIENT	STRENGTH	QUANTITY
Metoprolol tartarate tablets	100 mg	12
Ora-Plus:Ora-Sweet	1:1	
or Ora-Plus:Ora-Sweet SF		qs 120 mL

NOTE: In this study, the formulation was stored in amber clear plastic (polyethylene terephthalate) prescription ovals.

INSTRUCTIONS: Crush the tablets and triturate to a fine powder. Add approximately 20 mL of vehicle and levigate to a uniform paste. Add vehicle in geometric proportions almost to volume, mix thoroughly, and transfer to a graduate. Rinse the mortar with vehicle, add to the graduate, and qs to 120 mL.

NOTES

GENERIC NAME	**Metoprolol**
DOSAGE FORM	oral suspension
MADE FROM	tablets
CONCENTRATION	10 mg/mL
STABILITY	60 days
STABILITY REFERENCE	Allen LV Jr, et al. Am J Health Syst Pharm 1996; 53:2304-8.
STORE	refrigerate (preferable) or at room temperature
LABEL	shake well before use, refrigerate

INGREDIENT	STRENGTH	QUANTITY
Metoprolol tartarate tablets	100 mg	12
Cherry syrup (cherry syrup concentrate diluted 1:4 with simple syrup, NF)		qs 120 mL

NOTE: In this study, the formulation was stored in amber clear plastic (polyethylene terephthalate) prescription ovals.

INSTRUCTIONS: Crush the tablets and triturate to a fine powder. Add approximately 20 mL of vehicle and levigate to a uniform paste. Add vehicle in geometric proportions almost to volume, mix thoroughly, and transfer to a graduate. Rinse the mortar with vehicle, add to the graduate, and qs to 120 mL.

NOTES

Metronidazole

GENERIC NAME	Metronidazole
DOSAGE FORM	oral suspension
MADE FROM	powder
CONCENTRATION	50 mg/mL
STABILITY	60 days
STABILITY REFERENCE	Allen LV Jr, et al. Am J Health Syst Pharm 1996;53:2073-8
STORE	refrigerate (preferable) or at room temperature
LABEL	shake well before use, refrigerate

INGREDIENT	STRENGTH	QUANTITY
Metronidazole powder		6 g
Ora-Plus:Ora-Sweet or Ora-Plus:Ora-Sweet SF	1:1	aa qs 120 mL

NOTE: In this study, the formulation was stored in amber clear plastic (polyethylene terephthalate) prescription ovals.

INSTRUCTIONS: Weigh 6 g of metronidazole powder and place into a mortar. Add a small amount of the vehicle and mix to a uniform paste. Add vehicle in geometric proportions almost to volume. Transfer to a graduate and qs to 120 mL with vehicle while mixing.

NOTES

GENERIC NAME	**Metronidazole**
DOSAGE FORM	oral suspension
MADE FROM	tablets
CONCENTRATION	10 mg/mL
STABILITY	90 days
STABILITY REFERENCE	Mathew M, et al. J Clin Pharm Ther 1994;19:27-9
STORE	room temperature
LABEL	shake well before use, protect from light

INGREDIENT	STRENGTH	QUANTITY
Metronidazole (base) tablets	400 mg	3
or metronidazole base powder, USP		1200 mg
Ora-Plus		60 mL
Ora-Sweet		60 mL

NOTE: In this study, the formulation was stored in amber glass bottles.

INSTRUCTIONS: Triturate 3 tablets (or the powder) into a fine powder in a glass mortar. Mix Ora-Plus and Ora-Sweet in geometric proportions, with constant stirring, to produce 120 mL. Using 30 mL of this mixture, levigate the powder into a smooth suspension, adding the vehicle in geometric proportions. Transfer the suspension to a graduate. Rinse the mortar with sufficient vehicle into the graduate to bring the final volume to 120 mL.

NOTES

GENERIC NAME	**Metronidazole**
DOSAGE FORM	oral suspension
MADE FROM	powder
CONCENTRATION	50 mg/mL
STABILITY	60 days
STABILITY REFERENCE	Allen LV Jr, et al. Am J Health Syst Pharm 1996; 53:2073-8
STORE	refrigerate (preferable) or at room temperature
LABEL	shake well before use, refrigerate

INGREDIENT	STRENGTH	QUANTITY
Metronidazole powder		6 g
Cherry syrup (cherry syrup concentrate diluted 1:4 with simple syrup, NF)		qs 120 mL

NOTE: In this study, the formulation was stored in amber clear plastic (polyethylene terephthalate) prescription ovals.

INSTRUCTIONS: Weigh 6 g of the powder, triturate the powder and mix well. Add approximately 12 mL of vehicle and levigate to a uniform paste. Add vehicle in geometric proportions almost to volume, mix thoroughly, and transfer to a graduate. Rinse the mortar with vehicle, add to the graduate, and qs to 120 mL.

NOTES

GENERIC NAME	**Metronidazole**
DOSAGE FORM	oral suspension
MADE FROM	tablets
CONCENTRATION	15 mg/mL
STABILITY	60 days
STABILITY REFERENCE	Irwin DB, et al. Can J Hosp Pharm 1987;40:42-6
STORE	refrigerate
LABEL	shake well before use, refrigerate

INGREDIENT	STRENGTH	QUANTITY
Metronidazole tablets	250 mg	6
Water for irrigation		2 mL
[a]Chocolate–cherry syrup		qs 100 mL

[a]Artificial wild cherry flavor 0.12 mL, simple syrup, BP 60 mL, chocolate syrup (Nestle's Quik) qs 100 mL.

INSTRUCTIONS: Add the cherry flavor to the simple syrup, mixing well. Add the chocolate syrup to the cherry syrup and qs to 100 mL. Mix well. Crush the tablets into a fine powder. Add the water and levigate into a uniform paste. Add the chocolate–cherry syrup in geometric proportions, mix well, and transfer to a graduate. Rinse the mortar with more chocolate–cherry syrup, add to the graduate, and qs to 100 mL.

NOTES

GENERIC NAME	**Metronidazole Benzoate**
DOSAGE FORM	oral suspension
MADE FROM	tablets
CONCENTRATION	16 mg/mL
STABILITY	90 days
STABILITY REFERENCE	Mathew M, et al. J Clin Pharm Ther 1994;19:31-4
STORE	room temperature
LABEL	shake well before use

INGREDIENT	STRENGTH	QUANTITY
Metronidazole benzoate tablets	400 mg	4
Ora-Plus		50 mL
Ora-Sweet		50 mL

NOTE: In this study, the formulation was stored in amber glass bottles.

INSTRUCTIONS: Triturate 3 tablets into a fine powder in a glass mortar. Mix equal quantities of Ora-Plus and Ora-Sweet in geometric proportions, with constant stirring to produce 100 mL. Using 30 mL of this mixture, levigate the powder into a smooth suspension, adding the vehicle in geometric proportions. Transfer the suspension to a graduate. Rinse the mortar with sufficient vehicle into the graduate to bring the final volume to 100 mL.

NOTES

Metronidazole/Ceftizoxime

GENERIC NAME	Metronidazole/Ceftizoxime
DOSAGE FORM	injection
MADE FROM	injectables
CONCENTRATION	5 mg/mL and 10 mg/mL (ceftizoxime) (metronidazole)
STABILITY	see note
STABILITY REFERENCE	Nahata MC, et al. Am J Health Syst Pharm 1996; 53:1046-8
STORE	refrigerate
LABEL	expiration date, refrigerate

INGREDIENT	STRENGTH	QUANTITY
Ceftizoxime	10-g vial	1
Water for injection, USP		45 mL
Metronidazole injection	5 mg/mL	100 mL bag

NOTE: Both medications were stable for 10 days stored at 4 °C and for 10 days at 4 °C, then 48 hours at 25 °C. When stored at 25 °C, stability was maintained for only 3 days.

INSTRUCTIONS: In a laminar flow hood, add 45 mL of water for injection to a 10-g vial of ceftizoxime. Withdraw 5 mL of this solution and add to a 100-mL bag of ready-to-use metronidazole injection 5 mg/mL. The resulting solution contains 5 mg/mL metronidazole and 10 mg/mL ceftizoxime.

NOTES

GENERIC NAME	**Mexiletine**
DOSAGE FORM	oral suspension
MADE FROM	capsules
CONCENTRATION	10 mg/mL
STABILITY	28 days (4 °C); 14 days (25 °C)
STABILITY REFERENCE	Nahata MC, et al. J Am Pharm Assoc 2000;40: 257-9
STORE	refrigerate
LABEL	shake well before use, refrigerate

INGREDIENT	STRENGTH	QUANTITY
Mexiletine capsules	150 mg	8
Sorbitol solution, USP	70%	qs 120 mL

NOTE: In this study, the formulation was stored in amber plastic prescription bottles.

INSTRUCTIONS: Empty the contents of the capsules into a mortar and reduce to a fine powder. Add a small amount of the sorbital solution to the mortar and levigate to a fine paste. Add geometric proportions of the vehicle almost to volume. Transfer to a graduate and qs to 120 mL with vehicle. Stir well.

NOTES

GENERIC NAME	**Mexiletine**
DOSAGE FORM	oral suspension
MADE FROM	capsules
CONCENTRATION	10 mg/mL
STABILITY	91 days (4 °C); 70 days (25 °C)
STABILITY REFERENCE	Nahata MC, et al. J Am Pharm Assoc 2000;40: 257-9
STORE	refrigerate
LABEL	shake well before use, refrigerate

INGREDIENT	STRENGTH	QUANTITY
Mexiletine capsules	150 mg	8
Distilled water		qs 120 mL

NOTE: In this study, the formulation was stored in amber plastic prescription bottles.

INSTRUCTIONS: Empty the contents of the capsules into a mortar and reduce to a fine powder. Add a small amount of water and levigate to a uniform paste. Add water in geometric proportions and mix well. Transfer to a graduate, rinse the mortar with water, transfer the rinsings to the graduate, and qs to 120 mL. Stir well.

NOTES

GENERIC NAME	**Midazolam**
DOSAGE FORM	oral solution
MADE FROM	injection
CONCENTRATION	2.5 mg/mL
STABILITY	56 days (7 °C, 20 °C, 40 °C)
STABILITY REFERENCE	Steedman SL, et al. Am J Hosp Pharm 1992;49: 615-8
STORE	refrigerate (preferable) or at room temperature
LABEL	refrigerate

INGREDIENT	STRENGTH	QUANTITY
Midazolam HCl injection	5 mg/mL	60 mL
Simple syrup, NF		qs 120 mL

NOTE: In this study, the formulation was prepared using Syrpalta, a commercially available flavored, dye-free syrup. In this study, the formulation was stored in amber glass containers. Commercially available as a syrup, 2 mg/mL.

INSTRUCTIONS: Withdraw the midazolam HCl injection solution from the vial with a 50-mL syringe and needle. Add to a graduate and qs to volume with syrup. Mix well.

NOTES

GENERIC NAME	**Midazolam**
DOSAGE FORM	oral solution
MADE FROM	injection
CONCENTRATION	0.64 mg/mL, 0.35 mg/mL, 1.03 mg/mL
STABILITY	102 days
STABILITY REFERENCE	Walker SE, et al. Anesth Prog 1997;44:17-22
STORE	room temperature

INGREDIENT	STRENGTH	QUANTITY
Midazolam hydrochloride injection	5 mg/mL	qs to obtain the required concentration
[a]Orange-flavored syrup		qs to obtain the required concentration

[a]Simple syrup, NF 50 mL, pure orange extract 0.12 mL, red food coloring 1 drop, yellow food coloring 1 drop, distilled water qs to 100 mL

NOTE: In this study, the formulation was stored in high-density polyethylene containers. Commercially available as a syrup, 2 mg/mL.

INSTRUCTIONS: Add 30 mL of distilled water to 50 mL of simple syrup, then add the orange extract and food coloring with shaking. Add more distilled water and qs to 100 mL. Mix appropriate amounts of the midazolam HCl injection solution and orange-flavored syrup to obtain the necessary concentration.

NOTES

GENERIC NAME	**Midazolam**
DOSAGE FORM	flavored gelatin
MADE FROM	injection
CONCENTRATION	1 mg/mL
STABILITY	28 days (−20 °C); 14 days (4 °C)
STABILITY REFERENCE	Bhatt-Mehta V, et al. Am J Hosp Pharm 1993; 50:472-5
STORE	refrigerate or freeze
LABEL	refrigerate or freeze

INGREDIENT	STRENGTH	QUANTITY
Midazolam hydrochloride injection	5 mg/mL	45 mL
Tropical fruit punch–flavored gelatin (Jell-O)	3 oz	1 box
Distilled water		180 mL

NOTE: In this study, the formulation was stored in plastic medicine cups. Commercially available as a syrup, 2 mg/mL.

INSTRUCTIONS: Heat the distilled water to boiling in a beaker on a hot plate. Add 1 small box of tropical fruit punch–flavored gelatin to the water and stir until the particles dissolve. Allow the solution to cool to 40 °C. The initial pH of the gelatin solution should be approximately 4.0. Add 45 mL of midazolam HCl injection solution (5 mg/mL) to the cooled gelatin solution and stir well. Transfer 5-mL portions of this gelatin solution to unit-dose plastic medicine cups. Refrigerate the cups until the gelatin solution is firm (1–2 h). Place the cups in a food storage bag and store in the refrigerator or the freezer.

NOTES

GENERIC NAME	**Midazolam**
DOSAGE FORM	flavored gelatin
MADE FROM	injection
CONCENTRATION	2 mg/mL
STABILITY	28 days (–20 °C); 14 days (4 °C)
STABILITY REFERENCE	Bhatt-Mehta V, et al. Am J Hosp Pharm 1993; 50:472-5
STORE	refrigerate or freeze
LABEL	refrigerate or freeze

INGREDIENT	STRENGTH	QUANTITY
Midazolam hydrochloride injection	5 mg/mL	90 mL
Tropical fruit punch–flavored gelatin (Jell-O)	3 oz	1 box
Distilled water		135 mL

NOTE: In this study, the formulation was stored in plastic medicine cups. Commercially available as a syrup, 2 mg/mL.

INSTRUCTIONS: Heat the distilled water to boiling in a beaker on a hot plate. Add 1 small box of tropical fruit punch–flavored gelatin to the water and stir until the particles dissolve. Allow the solution to cool to 40 °C. The initial pH of the gelatin solution should be approximately 4.0. Add 45 mL of midazolam HCl injection solution (5 mg/mL) to the cooled gelatin solution and stir well. Transfer 5-mL portions of this gelatin solution to unit-dose plastic medicine cups. Refrigerate the cups until the gelatin solution is firm (1–2 h). Place the cups in a food storage bag and store in the refrigerator or the freezer.

NOTES

GENERIC NAME	**Mitomycin**
DOSAGE FORM	ophthalmic drops
MADE FROM	injection
CONCENTRATION	0.5 mg/mL
STABILITY	14 days (4 °C); 7 days (25 °C)
STABILITY REFERENCE	Fiscella RG, et al. Am J Hosp Pharm 1992;49:2440
STORE	refrigerate
LABEL	refrigerate, for ophthalmic use only

INGREDIENT	STRENGTH	QUANTITY
Mitomycin injection	5 mg	vial
Sterile water for injection		10 mL

NOTE: Sterility testing not performed.

INSTRUCTIONS: Reconstitute the vial with sterile water for injection to achieve a concentration of 0.5 mg/mL using aseptic technique. Withdraw the liquid and dispense into a sterile ophthalmic dropper bottle. American Society of Health-System Pharmacists' guidelines (Am J Hosp Pharm 1993;50:1462-3) for compounding ophthalmic products should be considered while preparing this formulation.

NOTES

GENERIC NAME	**Morphine**
DOSAGE FORM	oral solution
MADE FROM	elixir
CONCENTRATION	0.2 mg/mL
STABILITY	60 days
STABILITY REFERENCE	Nahata MC, et al. Presented at: American Society of Health-System Pharmacists Midyear Clinical Meeting, 2007 (poster)
STORE	room temperature
LABEL	protect from light

INGREDIENT	STRENGTH	QUANTITY
Morphine sulfate elixir	10 mg/5 mL	5 mL
Distilled water		50 mL

NOTE: This formulation was stored in amber oral syringes.
INSTRUCTIONS: Dilute 5 mL of morphine sulfate elixir (10 mg/5 mL) by adding 45 mL of distilled water to make a final volume of 50 mL. Mix well. The solution can be drawn into amber oral syringes, capped, and stored for use.

NOTES

GENERIC NAME	**Morphine Sulfate**
DOSAGE FORM	injection
MADE FROM	injection
CONCENTRATION	1 mg/mL
STABILITY	91 days
STABILITY REFERENCE	Nahata MC, et al. Am J Hosp Pharm 1992;49: 2785-7
STORE	refrigerate
LABEL	refrigerate

INGREDIENT	STRENGTH	QUANTITY
Morphine sulfate tubex	10 mg/mL	0.5 mL
Bacteriostatic NaCl 0.9%		4.5 mL

NOTE: Use for neonatal doses.
INSTRUCTIONS: Mix in an empty sterile vial.

NOTES

GENERIC NAME	**Moxifloxacin**
DOSAGE FORM	oral suspension
MADE FROM	tablets
CONCENTRATION	20 mg/mL
STABILITY	90 days
STABILITY REFERENCE	Hutchinson DJ, et al. Am J Health Syst Pharm 2009;66:665-7
STORE	room temperature
LABEL	shake well before use, protect from light

INGREDIENT	STRENGTH	QUANTITY
Moxifloxacin tablets	400 mg	3
Ora-Plus		30 mL
Ora-Sweet or Ora-Sweet SF		30 mL

NOTE:	In this study, the formulation was stored in amber child-resistant prescription bottles.
INSTRUCTIONS:	Triturate 3 tablets into a fine powder in a glass mortar. Mix equal quantities of Ora-Plus and Ora-Sweet in geometric proportions, with constant stirring, to produce 60 mL. Using 30 mL of this mixture, levigate the powder into a smooth suspension, adding the vehicle in geometric proportions. Transfer the suspension into a 2-oz child-resistant amber prescription bottle. Rinse the mortar with sufficient vehicle into the bottle to bring the final volume to 60 mL.

NOTES

GENERIC NAME	**Mupirocin**
DOSAGE FORM	topical
MADE FROM	ointment
CONCENTRATION	1% w/w
STABILITY	refer to table
STABILITY REFERENCE	Jagota NK, et al. J Clin Pharm Ther 1992;17:181-4
STORE	room temperature (37 °C)
LABEL	for external use only

INGREDIENT	STRENGTH	QUANTITY
Mupirocin ointment	2%	15 g
[a]Commercial topical product	15 g	

Stability of mupirocin in various commercial topical products at 37 °C:

Hibiclens liquid soap 60 days
Nizoral cream 30 days[a]
Kenalog cream 15 days
Kenalog ointment 30 days
Lotrimin cream 45 days[a]
Lotrimin solution 60 days

Hytone cream 45 days[a]
Hytone ointment 45 days[a]
Valisone ointment 60 days[a]
Vytone cream 60 days[a]
Silvadene cream 45 days

[a]Product may separate into two layers, but will become homogenous upon remixing.

NOTE:	In this study, the formulation was stored in glass ointment jars. Stability-indicating analytical methods not used.
INSTRUCTIONS:	Accurately weigh equal quantities (15 g) of the mupirocin ointment 2% and the desired commercial topical product. Thoroughly mix the two in geometric proportions into a smooth ointment on a porcelain pill tile using a plastic spatula. Transfer the product to an ointment jar.

NOTES

Mycophenolate

GENERIC NAME	Mycophenolate
DOSAGE FORM	oral suspension
MADE FROM	capsules
CONCENTRATION	50 mg/mL
STABILITY	210 days
STABILITY REFERENCE	Venkataramanan R, et al. Ann Pharmacother 1998;32:755-7
STORE	refrigerate
LABEL	shake well before use, use cytotoxic drug precautions, refrigerate

INGREDIENT	STRENGTH	QUANTITY
Mycophenolate mofetil capsules	250 mg	6
Ora-Plus		7.5 mL
Cherry syrup, USP		qs 30 mL

NOTE: Prepare under vertical flow hood. In this study, the formulation was stored in amber bottles. Commercially available as an oral powder for solution, 200 mg/mL.

INSTRUCTIONS: Empty contents of capsules into a glass mortar. Wet with Ora-Plus and levigate to a smooth paste. Add cherry syrup (~15 mL) in geometric proportions until suspension is pourable. Transfer suspension to a 50-mL graduate. Rinse the mortar with cherry syrup, add to the graduate, and qs to 30 mL.

NOTES

GENERIC NAME	**Mycophenolate**
DOSAGE FORM	oral suspension
MADE FROM	capsules
CONCENTRATION	100 mg/mL
STABILITY	28 days
STABILITY REFERENCE	Swenson CF, et al. Am J Health Syst Pharm 1999;56:2224-6
STORE	refrigerate
LABEL	shake well before use, use cytotoxic drug precautions, refrigerate

INGREDIENT	STRENGTH	QUANTITY
Mycophenolate mofetil capsules	250 mg	80
Artificial cherry flavoring		0.8 mL
FD&C red no. 40	10% w/v	0.1 mL
Ora-Plus		200 mL

NOTE: Prepare under vertical flow hood. In this study, the formulation was stored in amber polyethylene terephthalate glycol clear plastic bottles. Commercially available as an oral powder for solution, 200 mg/mL.

INSTRUCTIONS: Mix the artificial cherry flavoring and the coloring agent in geometric proportions in a glass mortar. Add Ora-Plus to this mixture in geometric proportions and prepare the vehicle for the suspension. Empty contents of capsules into a glass mortar. Wet with the liquid vehicle and levigate to a smooth paste. Add more vehicle (~50 mL) in geometric proportions until suspension is pourable. Transfer suspension to a 250-mL graduate. Rinse the mortar with more vehicle, add to the graduate, and qs to 200 mL.

NOTES

GENERIC NAME	**Mycophenolate**
DOSAGE FORM	oral suspension
MADE FROM	capsules
CONCENTRATION	100 mg/mL
STABILITY	121 days (2–8 °C and 23–25 °C)
STABILITY REFERENCE	Anaizi NH, et al. Am J Health Syst Pharm 1998; 55:926-9
STORE	refrigerate (preferable) or at room temperature
LABEL	shake well before use, use cytotoxic drug precautions, refrigerate

INGREDIENT	STRENGTH	QUANTITY
Mycophenolate mofetil capsules	250 mg	80
Sterile water for irrigation, USP		qs
Cherry syrup, USP		qs 200 mL

NOTE:	Prepare under vertical flow hood. In this study, the formulation was stored in amber polyethylene terephthalate glycol bottles. Commercially available as an oral powder for solution, 200 mg/mL.
INSTRUCTIONS:	Empty contents of capsules into a glass mortar. Wet with a sufficient quantity of sterile water for irrigation, USP, and levigate to a smooth paste. Add cherry syrup (~50 mL) in geometric proportions until suspension is pourable. Transfer suspension to a 250-mL graduate. Rinse the mortar with cherry syrup, add to the graduate, and qs to 200 mL.

NOTES

GENERIC NAME	**Nadolol**
DOSAGE FORM	oral suspension
MADE FROM	tablets
CONCENTRATION	10 mg/mL
STABILITY	30 days
STABILITY REFERENCE	experience
STORE	refrigerate
LABEL	refrigerate, shake well before use

INGREDIENT	STRENGTH	QUANTITY
Nadolol tablets	80 mg	10
Ora-Plus		70 mL
Ora-Sweet		

NOTE:
INSTRUCTIONS: The formulation was stored in amber prescription bottles. Mix Ora-Plus and Ora-Sweet in geometric proportions to make the vehicle. Place the tablets in a glass mortar and triturate to a fine powder. Levigate the powder with minimal amount of the vehicle to produce a smooth suspension. Add the vehicle in geometric proportions and mix well. Transfer to graduate. Rinse mortar with small amounts of vehicle and add to graduate to make up the final volume to 80 mL.

NOTES

GENERIC NAME	**Naratriptan**
DOSAGE FORM	oral suspension
MADE FROM	tablets
CONCENTRATION	0.5 mg/mL
STABILITY	90 days
STABILITY REFERENCE	Zhang YP, et al. Int J Pharmaceut Compd 2000; 4:69-71
STORE	refrigerate
LABEL	shake well before use, refrigerate

INGREDIENT	STRENGTH	QUANTITY
Naratriptan tablets	2.5 mg	50
Ora-Plus:Ora-Sweet or Ora-Plus:Ora-Sweet SF	1:1	qs 250 mL

INSTRUCTIONS: Crush tablets in a mortar and reduce to a fine powder. Add 125 mL of Ora-Plus to the powder in small amounts, mixing well after each addition. Transfer the mixture to a graduate, rinse the mortar, then qs with Ora-Sweet or Ora-Sweet SF to a total of 250 mL while mixing.

NOTES

GENERIC NAME	**Nifedipine**
DOSAGE FORM	oral suspension
MADE FROM	capsules
CONCENTRATION	4 mg/mL
STABILITY	90 days
STABILITY REFERENCE	Nahata MC, et al. J Am Pharm Assoc 2002;42: 865-7
STORE	refrigerate (preferable) or at room temperature
LABEL	shake well before use, refrigerate

INGREDIENT	STRENGTH	QUANTITY
Nifedipine capsules to obtain liquid equivalent to 400 mg		400 mg
[a]Methylcellulose with parabens	1%	7 mL
Simple syrup, NF		qs 100 mL

[a]See methylcellulose oral suspension

NOTE:	In this study, the formulation was stored in plastic prescription bottles.
INSTRUCTIONS:	Withdraw nifedipine liquid from the capsules using a needle and a syringe. Measure the required amount of liquid and add to a mortar. Add methylcellulose gel in geometric proportions and mix well. Add simple syrup in geometric proportions with constant mixing and transfer to a graduate. Rinse the mortar with syrup, transfer to the graduate, and qs to 100 mL.

NOTES

GENERIC NAME	**Nifedipine**
DOSAGE FORM	oral suspension
MADE FROM	tablets
CONCENTRATION	1 mg/mL
STABILITY	28 days
STABILITY REFERENCE	Helin-Tanninen M, et al. Clin Pharm Ther 2001; 26:59-66
STORE	refrigerate (preferable) or at room temperature
LABEL	shake well before use, refrigerate

INGREDIENT	STRENGTH	QUANTITY
Nifedipine tablets	10 mg	5
[a]Hydroxypropylmethyl-cellulose solution	1%	qs 50 mL

[a]See hydroxypropylmethylcellulose solution

NOTE: Refer to hydroxypropylmethylcellulose solution for preparation. Stability-indicating analytical methods not used.

INSTRUCTIONS: Triturate the tablets in a glass mortar to a fine powder. Add a small amount of the hydroxypropylmethylcellulose solution and soak for ~5 minutes to dissolve the tablet coating. Levigate to a uniform paste. Add vehicle in geometric proportions almost to volume and levigate. Transfer to a graduate and qs to 50 mL.

NOTES

GENERIC NAME	**Nifedipine**
DOSAGE FORM	oral suspension
MADE FROM	capsules
CONCENTRATION	4 mg/mL
STABILITY	90 days
STABILITY REFERENCE	Nahata MC, et al. J Am Pharm Assoc 2002;42: 865-7
STORE	refrigerate (preferable) or at room temperature
LABEL	shake well before use, refrigerate

INGREDIENT	STRENGTH	QUANTITY
Nifedipine capsules to obtain liquid equivalent to 400 mg		400 mg
Ora-Plus		
Ora-Sweet		aa qs 100 mL

NOTE: In this study, the formulation was stored in plastic prescription bottles.

INSTRUCTIONS: Withdraw nifedipine liquid from the capsules using a needle and a syringe. Measure the required amount of liquid and add to a mortar. Add a 1:1 mixture of Ora-Plus and Ora-Sweet in geometric proportions and mix well. Transfer the suspension to a graduate, rinse the mortar with vehicle, transfer to graduate, and qs to 100 mL.

NOTES

GENERIC NAME	**Nifedipine**
DOSAGE FORM	oral solution
MADE FROM	capsules
CONCENTRATION	10 mg/mL
STABILITY	35 days when stored in amber glass bottles; 14 days when stored in amber oral syringes wrapped in aluminum foil
STABILITY REFERENCE	Dentinger PJ, et al. Am J Health Syst Pharm 2003;60:1019-22
STORE	room temperature
LABEL	protect from light

INGREDIENT	STRENGTH	QUANTITY
Nifedipine powder		3.2 g
Polyethylene glycol 400		190 mL
Glycerin		127 mL
Peppermint oil		3.2 mL

NOTE: In this study, the formulation was stored in amber glass bottles and amber oral syringes wrapped in aluminum foil.

INSTRUCTIONS: To a suitable-sized glass beaker, add the polyethylene glycol 400. Add the nifedipine powder, with constant stirring, using a glass rod or Teflon-coated stir bar, if available. Add the glycerin to this mixture with stirring. Heat the cloudy yellow liquid to approximately 95 °C, stirring constantly and maintaining the temperature as all of the nifedipine goes into solution. Filter the hot clear solution through a 1.2-μm glass microfiber filter and continue stirring until the liquid cools to room temperature. Add the peppermint oil to the cool liquid.

NOTES

GENERIC NAME	**Nizatidine**
DOSAGE FORM	oral suspension
MADE FROM	capsules
CONCENTRATION	2.5 mg/mL
STABILITY	2 days
STABILITY REFERENCE	Lantz MD, et al. Am J Hosp Pharm 1990;47: 2716-9
STORE	refrigerate
LABEL	shake well before use, refrigerate

INGREDIENT	STRENGTH	QUANTITY
Nizatidine capsule	300 mg	1
Gatorade Thirst Quencher lemon lime or Ocean Spray Cran-Grape grape cranberry drink or Speas Farm apple juice or V8 100% vegetable juice		120 mL

INSTRUCTIONS: Add the contents of a capsule equivalent to 300 mg to 120 mL of one of the above vehicles and shake gently.

NOTES

Norfloxacin

GENERIC NAME	**Norfloxacin**
DOSAGE FORM	oral suspension
MADE FROM	tablets
CONCENTRATION	20 mg/mL
STABILITY	56 days
STABILITY REFERENCE	Johnson CE, et al. Am J Health Syst Pharm 2001;58:577-9
STORE	refrigerate (preferable) or at room temperature
LABEL	shake well before use, refrigerate

INGREDIENT	STRENGTH	QUANTITY
Norfloxacin tablets	400 mg	3
Ora-Plus:strawberry syrup		qs 60 mL

NOTE: In this study, the formulation was stored in amber plastic prescription bottles. Strawberry syrup was prepared by mixing 3200 mL of simple syrup, NF, with 600 mL of Strawberry Fountain Syrup (Gordon Food Services, Grand Rapids, MI).

INSTRUCTIONS: Triturate the tablets in a glass mortar and pestle to a fine powder. Add a small amount of the vehicle and levigate it to a smooth paste. Add a sufficient amount (~30 mL) of the vehicle in geometric proportions to obtain a uniform mixture. Transfer the mixture to a graduate. Rinse the mortar and pestle repeatedly with the remaining vehicle, add to the graduate, and qs to 60 mL.

NOTES

GENERIC NAME	**Omeprazole**
DOSAGE FORM	oral suspension
MADE FROM	capsules
CONCENTRATION	2 mg/mL
STABILITY	30 days (at 5 °C and –20 °C)
STABILITY REFERENCE	Quercia RA, et al. Am J Health Syst Pharm 1997; 54:1833-6
STORE	refrigerate or freeze
LABEL	shake well before use, refrigerate or freeze

INGREDIENT	STRENGTH	QUANTITY
Omeprazole capsules	20 mg	5
Sodium bicarbonate injection, USP	8.4%	50 mL

INSTRUCTIONS: Pull out the plunger from a 60-mL luer-lok syringe and attach an 18-gauge needle. Empty the contents of the capsules in the syringe and replace the plunger. Draw up 50 mL of sodium bicarbonate 8.4% injection solution from a vial. Replace the needle with a fluid-dispensing connector and attach another 60-mL syringe to the fluid-dispensing connector. Gently transfer the contents of the syringe back and forth until the granules completely dissolve. Transfer the solution to one of the syringes, disconnect the empty syringe, and replace the fluid-containing syringe with an 18-gauge needle. Transfer the solution to an empty vial.

NOTES

GENERIC NAME	**Omeprazole**
DOSAGE FORM	oral suspension
MADE FROM	capsules
CONCENTRATION	2 mg/mL
STABILITY	45 days
STABILITY REFERENCE	DiGiacinto JL, et al. Ann Pharmacother 2000;34:600-5
STORE	refrigerate
LABEL	shake well before use, refrigerate

INGREDIENT	STRENGTH	QUANTITY
Omeprazole capsules	20 mg	10
Sodium bicarbonate injection, USP	8.4%	100 mL

NOTE: In this study, the formulation was stored in amber plastic oral syringes.

INSTRUCTIONS: Empty contents of the capsules into a 250-mL Erlenmeyer flask. Measure 100 mL of sodium bicarbonate solution in a graduate and add to the flask. Stir the mixture with a magnetic stirrer for 30 minutes.

NOTES

GENERIC NAME	**Ondansetron**
DOSAGE FORM	oral suspension
MADE FROM	injection
CONCENTRATION	0.84 mg/mL
STABILITY	7 days
STABILITY REFERENCE	Graham CL, et al. Am J Hosp Pharm 1993;50: 106-8
STORE	refrigerate (preferable) or at room temperature
LABEL	shake well before use, refrigerate

INGREDIENT	STRENGTH	QUANTITY
Ondansetron hydrochloride injection	2 mg/mL	168 mL
Cherry		231 mL

NOTE: In this study, the formulation was stored in amber plastic bottles. Commercially available as an oral solution, 4 mg/5 mL, and orally disintegrating tablets, 4 mg and 8 mg.

INSTRUCTIONS: Mix the two solutions in geometric proportions.

NOTES

GENERIC NAME	**Ondansetron**
DOSAGE FORM	oral suspension
MADE FROM	tablets
CONCENTRATION	0.8 mg/mL
STABILITY	42 days
STABILITY REFERENCE	Williams CL, et al. Am J Hosp Pharm 1994;51:806-8
STORE	refrigerate
LABEL	shake well before use, refrigerate

INGREDIENT	STRENGTH	QUANTITY
Ondansetron hydrochloride tablets	8 mg	10
Ora-Plus		50 mL
Ora-Sweet or Ora-Sweet SF		qs 100 mL

NOTE: In this study, the formulation was stored in amber plastic bottles. Commercially available as an oral solution, 4 mg/5 mL, and orally disintegrating tablets, 4 mg and 8 mg.

INSTRUCTIONS: Crush the tablets and triturate to a fine powder in a mortar. Flaking of the tablet coating may occur. The fine powder is thoroughly levigated with Ora-Plus in increments of 5 mL until a smooth paste is formed. The vehicle is then added in geometric proportions. Transfer the suspension to a graduate. Rinse the mortar with vehicle, add to the graduate, and qs to 100 mL.

NOTES

Oral Preoperative Sedative

GENERIC NAME	
DOSAGE FORM	oral solution
MADE FROM	liquid
CONCENTRATION	atropine 0.024 mg/promethazine syrup 1.85 mg/chloral hydrate 60 mg/mL
STABILITY	6 months
STABILITY REFERENCE	experience
STORE	room temperature, in amber glass bottles

INGREDIENT	STRENGTH	QUANTITY
Atropine solution	1 mg/mL	72 mL
Promethazine syrup	25 mg/5 mL	1110 mL
Chloral hydrate syrup	500 mg/5 mL	1800 mL
Purified water, USP		18 mL

NOTE: To make atropine stock solution, add 150 mg atropine sulfate powder to a graduate and qs to 150 mL with water. Store in an amber glass bottle and label for compounding use only — do not dispense. Have atropine weight checked by a pharmacist before mixing. Dose for full solution: 2 mL/10 lb. Maximum dose: 25 mL.

INSTRUCTIONS: Mix the ingredients in a 1-gallon container.

NOTES

GENERIC NAME	**Oseltamivir**
DOSAGE FORM	oral suspension
MADE FROM	capsules
CONCENTRATION	15 mg/mL
STABILITY	35 days refrigerated, 13 days room temperature
STABILITY REFERENCE	Winiarski AP, et al. J Am Pharm Assoc (2003) 2007;47:747-55
STORE	refrigerate (relative humidity 60% ± 5%) (preferable); room temperature (relative humidity 65% ± 5%)
LABEL	shake well before use, refrigerate

INGREDIENT	STRENGTH	QUANTITY
Oseltamivir capsules	75 mg	12
Cherry syrup		qs 60 mL

NOTE: In this study, the formulation was stored in amber glass and polyethylene terephthalate bottles..

INSTRUCTIONS: Empty the contents of 12 capsules into a glass mortar and triturate into a fine powder. Add one third of the cherry syrup in geometric proportions and triturate into a smooth suspension. Transfer the suspension to the required container. Rinse mortar with cherry syrup and transfer into the bottle, to bring the final volume to 60 mL.

NOTES

GENERIC NAME	**Oseltamivir**
DOSAGE FORM	ooral suspension
MADE FROM	capsules
CONCENTRATION	15 mg/mL
STABILITY	35 days refrigerated, 13 days room temperature
STABILITY REFERENCE	Winiarski AP, et al. J Am Pharm Assoc (2003) 2007;47:747-55
STORE	refrigerate (relative humidity 60% ± 5%) (preferable); room temperature (relative humidity 65% ± 5%)
LABEL	shake well before use, rerigerate

INGREDIENT	STRENGTH	QUANTITY
Oseltamivir capsules	75 mg	12
Ora-Sweet SF		qs 60 mL

NOTE: In this study, the formulation was stored in amber glass and polyethyleneterephthalate bottles.

INSTRUCTIONS: Empty the contents of 12 capsules in a glass mortar and triturate into a fine powder. Add one third of Ora-Sweet SF in geometric proportions and triturate into a smooth suspension. Transfer the suspension to the required container. Rinse mortar with Ora-Sweet SF and transfer into the bottle to bring the final volume in the bottle to 60 mL.

NOTES

GENERIC NAME	**Penicillamine**
DOSAGE FORM	oral suspension
MADE FROM	capsules
CONCENTRATION	50 mg/mL
STABILITY	35 days
STABILITY REFERENCE	deCastro FJ, et al. Hosp Pharm 1977;12:446-8
STORE	refrigerate
LABEL	shake well before use, refrigerate

INGREDIENT	STRENGTH	QUANTITY
Penicillamine capsules	250 mg	60
[a]Spray-dried cherry imitation flavor powder		3 g
Carboxymethylcellulose sodium		3 g
Sucrose		150 g
Citric acid		0.300 g
Methylparaben		0.360 g
Propylparaben		0.060 g
Distilled water		qs 300 mL (added only at time of dispensing)

[a]Available as Aromalok by Fritsche, Dodge and Olcott, Inc., 76 Ninth Ave., New York, NY 10011, and Beck Flavors, 1403–1405 State St., East St. Louis, IL 62205.

NOTE: Stability-indicating analytical methods not used.
INSTRUCTIONS: Triturate the contents of the capsules to make a uniform mixture. Add carboxymethylcellulose, sweeteners, flavoring agents, and preservatives in geometric proportions and mix well. Add distilled water and qs to 300 mL just before dispensing the formulation.

NOTES

GENERIC NAME	**Pentoxifylline**
DOSAGE FORM	oral suspension
MADE FROM	tablets
CONCENTRATION	20 mg/mL
STABILITY	91 days
STABILITY REFERENCE	Abdel-Rahman S, et al. Am J Health Syst Pharm 1997;54:1301-3
STORE	refrigerate (preferable) or at room temperature
LABEL	shake well before use, refrigerate

INGREDIENT	STRENGTH	QUANTITY
Pentoxifylline tablets	400 mg	10
Purified water		qs 200 mL

NOTE: In this study, the formulation was stored in amber glass and plastic prescription bottles.

INSTRUCTIONS: Crush the tablets, including coating, in a wedgewood mortar and pestle. Triturate with a small amount of water to make a paste, then qs with water to the final concentration.

NOTES

GENERIC NAME	**Phenobarbital**
DOSAGE FORM	injection
MADE FROM	injection
CONCENTRATION	10 mg/mL
STABILITY	28 days
STABILITY REFERENCE	Nahata MC, et al. Am J Hosp Pharm 1986;43: 384-5
STORE	refrigerate in an empty sterile vial
LABEL	refrigerate

INGREDIENT	STRENGTH	QUANTITY
Phenobarbital injection	65 mg/mL	2 mL
Bacteriostatic water for injection		11 mL

INSTRUCTIONS: Mix in a sterile syringe.

NOTES

GENERIC NAME	**Phenobarbital**
DOSAGE FORM	oral solution
MADE FROM	powder
CONCENTRATION	3 mg/mL
STABILITY	30 days
STABILITY REFERENCE	Woods DJ. www.pharminfotech.co.nz/emixt
STORE	refrigerate, protect from light
LABEL	refrigerate, protect from light

INGREDIENT	STRENGTH	QUANTITY
Phenobarbitone sodium		300 mg
Glycerin		20 mL
Sorbitol		30 mL
[a]Parabens		0.1%
Water		qs 100 mL

[a]Methyl hydroxybenzoate 4 g, propyl hydroxybenzoate 1 g, propylene glycol qs 100 mL. Mix 2 mL of this solution to 100 mL of formulation to give 0.1% parabens.

NOTE:	Sorbitol may be unacceptable to the patient or unavailable. Omitting this agent is unlikely to compromise short-term stability. If sorbitol is left out, increase the glycerin content from 20% to 40% (i.e., to 40 mL/100 mL). Phenobarbitone sodium solutions are susceptible to precipitation, especially if the pH drops to <8.5–9. Acidic flavors and syrups should not be added. If possible, check the final pH. Stability-indicating analytical methods not used. Commercially available as an elixir 15 mg/5 mL and 20 mg/5 mL.
INSTRUCTIONS:	Dissolve phenobarbitone in ~5 mL of water. Mix with glycerin and sorbitol in geometric proportions. Add the parabens solution. Transfer to a graduate, rinse the mortar with water, and add to graduate to qs to 100 mL. Mix well.

NOTES

GENERIC NAME	**Phenobarbital**
DOSAGE FORM	oral suspension
MADE FROM	tablets
CONCENTRATION	10 mg/mL
STABILITY	90 days
STABILITY REFERENCE	Cober MP, et al. Am J Health Syst Pharm 2007;64:644-6
STORE	room temperature
LABEL	shake well before use

INGREDIENT	STRENGTH	QUANTITY
Phenobarbital tablets	60 mg	10
Ora-Plus		30 mL
Ora-Sweet		30 mL

NOTE: In this study, the formulation was stored in amber child-resistant prescription bottles.

INSTRUCTIONS: Triturate 10 tablets into a fine powder in a glass mortar. Mix equal quantities of Ora-Plus and Ora-Sweet in geometric proportions, with constant stirring, to produce 60 mL. Using 15 mL of this mixture, levigate the powder into a smooth suspension, adding the vehicle in geometric proportions. Transfer the suspension to a 2-oz child-resistant amber prescription bottle. Rinse the mortar with sufficient vehicle into the bottle to bring the final volume to 60 mL.

NOTES

GENERIC NAME	**Phenoxybenzamine**
DOSAGE FORM	oral solution
MADE FROM	powder
CONCENTRATION	2 mg/mL
STABILITY	7 days
STABILITY REFERENCE	Lim LY, et al. Am J Health Syst Pharm 1997; 54:2073-8
STORE	refrigerate
LABEL	refrigerate

INGREDIENT	STRENGTH	QUANTITY
Phenoxybenzamine hydrochloride		200 mg
Propylene glycol		1 mL
Citric acid, USP		0.15 g
Distilled water		qs 100 mL

NOTE: In this study, the formulation was stored in amber glass prescription bottles.

INSTRUCTIONS: Dissolve phenoxybenzamine HCl in propylene glycol. Dissolve citric acid in a sufficient amount of water. Mix the two solutions in geometric proportions. Transfer to a 100-mL graduate and qs to 100 mL with distilled water.

NOTES

GENERIC NAME	**Phytonadione**
DOSAGE FORM	oral suspension
MADE FROM	tablets
CONCENTRATION	1 mg/mL
STABILITY	3 days
STABILITY REFERENCE	experience
STORE	refrigerate
LABEL	shake well before use, refrigerate

INGREDIENT	STRENGTH	QUANTITY
Phytonadione tablets	5 mg	6
Purified water, USP		5 mL
Methylcellulose	1%	5 mL
Sorbitol solution	70%	qs ad 30 mL

NOTE: Use no reducing agents.
INSTRUCTIONS: Triturate the tablets in a mortar. Add the water and methylcellulose while mixing. Transfer to a graduate, qs with sorbitol, and mix well.

NOTES

GENERIC NAME	**Phytonadione**
DOSAGE FORM	oral solution
MADE FROM	powder
CONCENTRATION	1 mg/mL
STABILITY	175 days
STABILITY REFERENCE	Sewell GJ, et al. J Clin Pharm Ther 1988;13:73-6
STORE	refrigerate
LABEL	refrigerate

INGREDIENT	STRENGTH	QUANTITY
Phytonadione		0.100 g
Cremophor EL		2 g
Water for injection		qs 100 mL

NOTE:	Administration of intravenous Cremophor EL has been associated with abnormal lipoprotein patterns, anaphylactoid reactions, alterations in blood viscosity, and erythrocyte aggregation. In this study, the formulation was stored in amber oral polypropylene syringes.
INSTRUCTIONS:	Mix phytonadione and Cremophor EL. Dilute the mixture gradually with water for injection to 100 mL. Sparge the solution with nitrogen for 3 minutes and sterilize by filtering through a 0.2-µm filter. Transfer aseptically to oral syringe.

NOTES

GENERIC NAME	**Pilocarpine**
DOSAGE FORM	oral solution
MADE FROM	ophthalmic drops
CONCENTRATION	3 mg/mL
STABILITY	90 days (4 °C); 60 days (25 °C)
STABILITY REFERENCE	Fawcett JP, et al. Int J Pharm Pract 1994;3:14-8
STORE	refrigerate (preferable) or at room temperature
LABEL	refrigerate, for ophthalmic use only

INGREDIENT	STRENGTH	QUANTITY
Pilocarpine eye drops	6%	15 mL (1 bottle 5 mL)
Glycerin		20 mL
ᵃMethyl hydroxybenzoate/ propyl hydroxybenzoate	0.1%	
Lemon spirit (optional)		0.1 mL
Sodium citrate		1.13 g
Citric acid monohydrate		0.27 g
Water		qs 100 mL

ᵃMethyl hydroxybenzoate 4 g, propyl hydroxybenzoate 1 g, propylene glycol qs 100 mL. Mix 2 mL of this solution with 100 mL of formulation to give 0.1% concentration.

NOTE:	Pilocarpine 6% eye drops contain pilocarpine HCl 60 mg/mL, hypromellose 3 mg/mL, benzalkonium chloride 0.1 mg/mL, and sodium edetate 0.5 mg/mL. It is preferable to check the final pH of this preparation and, if necessary, add 50–100 mg of citric acid to bring the pH within the approximate range of 4.5–5.5. In this study, the formulation was stored in amber high-density polyethylene bottles. Sterility testing not performed.
INSTRUCTIONS:	Dissolve the citric acid and sodium citrate in ~5 mL of water. Mix the eye drops solution, glycerin, and citric acid solution in geometric proportions. Add the parabens solution and lemon spirit and mix well. Transfer to a graduate and qs with water to 100 mL. Stir well.

NOTES

GENERIC NAME	**Potassium Perchlorate**
DOSAGE FORM	oral syrup
MADE FROM	crystals
CONCENTRATION	6.7 mg/mL
STABILITY	276 days
STABILITY REFERENCE	Williams CC. Am J Hosp Pharm 1977;34:93-5
STORE	room temperature

INGREDIENT	STRENGTH	QUANTITY
Potassium perchlorate		6.7 g
Distilled water		500 mL
Alcohol, USP		8.33 mL
Methylparabens		2.0 g
Propylparabens		0.20 g
[a]Imitation cherry syrup		qs 1000 mL

[a]Imitation cherry syrup is prepared by adding 7.8 mL of imitation cherry concentrate (Cino Chemical Co., Cincinnati, OH) to simple syrup, NF, and the volume is made up to 1000 mL.

NOTE: In this study, the formulation was stored in ground glass–stoppered vials. Refrigeration of this solution is not recommended since the salt forms crystals, which dissolve very slowly. Stability-indicating analytical methods not used.

INSTRUCTIONS: Dissolve potassium perchlorate in a 1000-mL glass flask with 500 mL of distilled water. Dissolve the parabens in alcohol in a separate flask and add to the perchlorate solution. Add the cherry syrup to this mixture with constant stirring and qs to 1000 mL.

NOTES

GENERIC NAME	**Pravastatin**
DOSAGE FORM	oral suspension
MADE FROM	tablets
CONCENTRATION	10 mg/mL
STABILITY	7 days
STABILITY REFERENCE	Nahata MC, et al. Presented at: American Society of Health-System Pharmacists Midyear Clinical Meeting, 2005
STORE	refrigerate (prefereable) or room temperature
LABEL	refrigerate, protect from light, shake well before use

INGREDIENT	STRENGTH	QUANTITY
Pravastatin tablets	40 mg	30
Simple syrup NF: 1% methylcellulose suspension	1:1	qs 120 mL

NOTE:	This formulation was stored in amber prescription bottles.
INSTRUCTIONS:	Mix simple syrup and 1% methylcellulose suspension thoroughly in a glass mortar, in geometric proportions, to prepare the vehicle. Triturate the tablets into a fine powder and levigate with a small proportion of the vehicle into a smooth suspension. Add vehicle in geometric proportions, with constant mixing. Transfer to a graduate. Rinse the mortar with a sufficient vehicle and transfer to the graduate to make up the final volume.

NOTES

GENERIC NAME	**Pravastatin**
DOSAGE FORM	oral suspension
MADE FROM	tablets
CONCENTRATION	10 mg/mL
STABILITY	7 days
STABILITY REFERENCE	Nahata MC, et al. Presented at: American Society of Health-System Pharmacists Midyear Clinical Meeting, 2005
STORE	refrigerate (preferable) or room temperature
LABEL	refrigerate, protect from light, shake well before use

INGREDIENT	STRENGTH	QUANTITY
Pravastatin tablets	40 mg	30
Ora-Plus:Ora-Sweet	1:1	qs 120 mL

NOTE: This formulation was stored in amber prescription bottles.

INSTRUCTIONS: Mix Ora-Plus and Ora-Sweet thoroughly, using a glass mortar and pestle, in geometric proportions, to prepare the vehicle. Triturate the tablets into a fine powder and levigate with a small proportion of the vehicle into a smooth suspension. Add the vehicle in geometric proportions with constant mixing. Transfer to a graduate. Rinse the mortar with sufficient vehicle and transfer to graduate to make up the final volume.

NOTES

GENERIC NAME	**Prednisolone**
DOSAGE FORM	oral solution
MADE FROM	powder
CONCENTRATION	0.5 mg/mL
STABILITY	92 days
STABILITY REFERENCE	Gupta VD. J Pharm Sci 1979;68:908-10
STORE	room temperature

INGREDIENT	STRENGTH	QUANTITY
Prednisolone		50 mg
Ethanol		10 mL
Sodium benzoate		0.1 g
Glycerin 50% aqueous solution or sorbitol 50% aqueous solution or sucrose 50% aqueous solution		qs 100 mL

NOTE: Stability-indicating analytical methods not used.
INSTRUCTIONS: Dissolve the prednisolone in ethanol. Dissolve sodium benzoate in ~10 mL of the vehicle. Mix the two solutions in geometric proportions and qs to 100 mL with the vehicle.

NOTES

GENERIC NAME	**Prednisone**
DOSAGE FORM	oral solution
MADE FROM	powder
CONCENTRATION	0.5 mg/mL
STABILITY	92 days
STABILITY REFERENCE	Gupta VD. J Pharm Sci 1979;68:908-10
STORE	room temperature

INGREDIENT	STRENGTH	QUANTITY
Prednisone		50 mg
Ethanol		10 mL
Sodium benzoate		0.1 g
Glycerin 50% aqueous solution		qs 100 mL

NOTE: Stability-indicating analytical methods not used.
INSTRUCTIONS: Dissolve the prednisone in ethanol. Dissolve sodium benzoate in ~10 mL of the vehicle. Mix the two solutions in geometric proportions and qs to 100 mL with the vehicle.

NOTES

GENERIC NAME	**Primaquine**
DOSAGE FORM	oral suspension
MADE FROM	tablets
CONCENTRATION	6-mg base/5 mL
STABILITY	7 days
STABILITY REFERENCE	experience
STORE	refrigerate
LABEL	shake well before use, refrigerate

INGREDIENT	STRENGTH	QUANTITY
Primaquine tablets	15-mg base	10
Carboxymethylcellulose	1.5%	10 mL
Simple syrup, NF		qs ad 125 mL

INSTRUCTIONS: Crush the tablets in a mortar and mix with small amounts of the carboxymethylcellulose solution until a smooth paste results. Add half of the syrup while mixing, transfer to a graduate, then qs to volume with syrup.

NOTES

GENERIC NAME	**Procainamide**
DOSAGE FORM	oral suspension
MADE FROM	capsules
CONCENTRATION	50 mg/mL
STABILITY	60 days
STABILITY REFERENCE	Allen LV Jr, et al. Am J Health Syst Pharm 1996;53:2073-8
STORE	refrigerate (preferable) or at room temperature
LABEL	shake well before use, refrigerate

INGREDIENT	STRENGTH	QUANTITY
Procainamide hydrochloride capsules	250 mg	24
Cherry syrup (cherry syrup concentrate diluted 1:4 with simple syrup, NF)		qs 120 mL

NOTE: In this study, the formulation was stored in amber clear plastic (polyethylene terephthalate) prescription ovals.

INSTRUCTIONS: Open capsules and place the powder into a mortar. Reduce to a fine powder. Add ~20 mL of vehicle and levigate to a uniform paste. Add vehicle in geometric proportions almost to volume, mix thoroughly, and transfer to a graduate. Rinse the mortar with vehicle, add to the graduate, and qs to 120 mL.

NOTES

GENERIC NAME	**Procainamide**
DOSAGE FORM	oral suspension
MADE FROM	capsules
CONCENTRATION	50 mg/mL
STABILITY	60 days
STABILITY REFERENCE	Allen LV Jr, et al. Am J Health Syst Pharm 1996;53:2073-8
STORE	refrigerate (preferable) or at room temperature
LABEL	shake well before use, refrigerate

INGREDIENT	STRENGTH	QUANTITY
Procainamide hydrochloride capsules	250 mg	24
Ora-Plus:Ora-Sweet or Ora-Plus:Ora-Sweet SF	1:1	qs 120 mL

NOTE: In this study, the formulation was stored in amber clear plastic (polyethylene terephthalate) prescription ovals.

INSTRUCTIONS: Open capsules and place the powder into a mortar. Reduce to a fine powder. Add ~20 mL of vehicle and levigate to a uniform paste. Add vehicle in geometric proportions almost to volume, mix thoroughly, and transfer to a graduate. Rinse the mortar with vehicle, add to the graduate, and qs to 120 mL.

NOTES

GENERIC NAME	**Procainamide**
DOSAGE FORM	oral suspension
MADE FROM	capsules
CONCENTRATION	50 mg/mL
STABILITY	456 days
STABILITY REFERENCE	Alexander KS, et al. Am J Hosp Pharm 1993;50: 693-8
STORE	room temperature
LABEL	shake well before use

INGREDIENT	STRENGTH	QUANTITY
Procainamide hydrochloride capsules	500 mg	50
Distilled water		165 mL
[a]Parabens		5 mL
Cherry flavoring		0.5 mL
Simple syrup, NF		qs 500 mL

[a]Methylparaben 10% w/v, propylparabens 2% w/v in propylene glycol.

NOTE:	In this study, the formulation was stored in amber-colored glass bottles.
INSTRUCTIONS:	Open capsules and place the powder into a mortar. Reduce to a fine powder. Add distilled water and levigate to a uniform paste. Add more water in geometric dilutions to form a uniform suspension. Add the parabens mixture and cherry flavoring and mix thoroughly. Add vehicle in geometric proportions, mix thoroughly, and transfer to a graduate. Rinse the mortar with vehicle, add to the graduate, and qs to 500 mL.

NOTES

GENERIC NAME	**Procainamide**
DOSAGE FORM	oral suspension
MADE FROM	capsules
CONCENTRATION	50 mg/mL
STABILITY	180 days (4–6 °C)
STABILITY REFERENCE	Alexander KS, et al. Am J Hosp Pharm 1993;50: 693-8
STORE	refrigerate
LABEL	shake well before use, refrigerate

INGREDIENT	STRENGTH	QUANTITY
Procainamide capsules	500 mg	50
Sterile water for irrigation, USP		25 mL
[a]Cherry syrup		qs 500 mL

[a]Sucrose 85% in distilled water, cherry flavoring 0.1%, 0.0005% FD&C red no. 40.

NOTE: pH should be at 6; there is usually no need to adjust the pH. In this study, the formulation was stored in amber bottles.

INSTRUCTIONS: Open capsules and place the powder into a mortar. Reduce to a fine powder. Add 25 mL of sterile water for irrigation, USP, and levigate to a uniform paste. Add 30 mL of vehicle in geometric proportions, mix thoroughly, and transfer to a graduate. Rinse the mortar with two 30-mL portions of the vehicle and add to the graduate. Add enough vehicle and qs to 500 mL.

NOTES

GENERIC NAME	**Procainamide**
DOSAGE FORM	oral suspension
MADE FROM	capsules
CONCENTRATION	100 mg/mL
STABILITY	180 days (4–6 °C)
STABILITY REFERENCE	Metras JI, et al. Am J Hosp Pharm 1992;49:1720-4
STORE	refrigerate
LABEL	shake well before use, refrigerate

INGREDIENT	STRENGTH	QUANTITY
Procainamide capsules	500 mg	100
Sterile water for irrigation, USP		25 mL
[a]Cherry syrup:methylcellulose 1%	30:70	qs 500 mL

[a]Sucrose 85% in distilled water, cherry flavoring 0.1%, 0.0005% FD&C red no. 40.

NOTE: Adjust the pH to 5 with 5M hydrochloric acid. In this study, the formulation was stored in amber bottles.

INSTRUCTIONS: Open capsules and place the powder into a mortar. Reduce to a fine powder. Add 25 mL of sterile water for irrigation, USP, and levigate to a uniform paste. Add 30 mL of vehicle in geometric proportions, mix thoroughly, and transfer to a graduate. Rinse the mortar twice with two 30-mL portions of the vehicle and add to the graduate. Add enough vehicle to qs to 500 mL.

NOTES

GENERIC NAME	**Procaine Hydrochloride**
DOSAGE FORM	injection
MADE FROM	powder
CONCENTRATION	100 mg/mL
STABILITY	11 months
STABILITY REFERENCE	experience
STORE	refrigerate
LABEL	refrigerate, for cardioplegic solution compounding

INGREDIENT	STRENGTH	QUANTITY
Procaine hydrochloride powder		100 g
Purified water for injection		qs ad 1000 mL

INSTRUCTIONS: Add the procaine hydrochloride powder to 800 mL of water and mix until dissolved, then qs to 1 L with water for injection. Filter through a 0.22-µm filter into 10-mL sterile glass syringes.

NOTES

GENERIC NAME	**Procarbazine Hydrochloride**
DOSAGE FORM	oral powder
MADE FROM	capsules
CONCENTRATION	5 mg/100 mg powder dilution
STABILITY	6 months
STABILITY REFERENCE	experience
STORE	room temperature

INGREDIENT	STRENGTH	QUANTITY
Procarbazine hydrochloride capsule	50 mg	1
Lactose		qs ad 1 g

INSTRUCTIONS: Empty the capsule into a mortar and triturate. Add small amounts of lactose powder and mix until uniform.

NOTES

Copyright © 2011 Harvey Whitney Books

GENERIC NAME	**Propranolol**
DOSAGE FORM	oral solution
MADE FROM	tablets
CONCENTRATION	5 mg/mL
STABILITY	84 days
STABILITY REFERENCE	Ahmed GH, et al. Aust J Hosp Pharm 1988;18: 312-8
STORE	refrigerate
LABEL	refrigerate, do not use if particulate matter seen, protect from light

INGREDIENT	STRENGTH	QUANTITY
Propranolol hydrochloride tablets	40 mg	12.5
Citric acid		1.0 g
Sodium benzoate		0.1 g
Cherry syrup BP		40 mL
Distilled water		qs 100 mL

NOTE: Discard the formulation if a precipitate develops. In this study, the formulation was stored in amber glass dispensing bottles. Stability-indicating analytical methods not used.
Commercially available as an oral solution, 4 mg/mL, 8 mg/mL, and 80 mg/mL.

INSTRUCTIONS: Dissolve citric acid in ~30 mL of distilled water. Dissolve sodium benzoate in a sufficient amount of distilled water. Crush and triturate the tablets into a fine powder. Disperse the powder with ~10 mL of the citric acid solution for ~10 minutes, preferably at 3000 rpm. Transfer the solution to an amber jar and shake for 1 hour. Filter the solution through a 0.22-μm Millipore filter. Wash the filter cake with two portions of 10 mL of the citric acid solution. Add the sodium benzoate solution and cherry syrup to the filtrate solution and mix. Add distilled water, qs to 100 mL, and continue mixing for at least another 20 minutes.

NOTES

GENERIC NAME	**Propylthiouracil**
DOSAGE FORM	oral suspension
MADE FROM	tablets
CONCENTRATION	5 mg/mL
STABILITY	91 days (4 °C); 70 days (25 °C)
STABILITY REFERENCE	Nahata MC, et al. Am J Health Syst Pharm 2000;57:1141-3
STORE	refrigerate
LABEL	shake well before use, refrigerate

INGREDIENT	STRENGTH	QUANTITY
Propylthiouracil tablets	50 mg	20
Ora-Plus		100 mL
Ora-Sweet		100 mL

NOTE: In this study, the formulation was stored in amber plastic prescription bottles.

INSTRUCTIONS: Crush the tablets in a mortar and reduce to a fine powder. Mix the two vehicles together. Add a small amount of the vehicle to the mortar and mix to a uniform paste. Add geometric amounts of vehicle while mixing. Transfer to a graduate and qs to volume while mixing.

NOTES

GENERIC NAME	**Propylthiouracil**
DOSAGE FORM	oral suspension
MADE FROM	tablets
CONCENTRATION	5 mg/mL
STABILITY	91 days (4 °C); 70 days (25 °C)
STABILITY REFERENCE	Nahata MC, et al. Am J Health Syst Pharm 2000; 57:1141-3
STORE	refrigerate
LABEL	shake well before use, refrigerate

INGREDIENT	STRENGTH	QUANTITY
Propylthiouracil tablets	50 mg	20
Methylcellulose solution 1%:simple syrup, NF	1:1	qs 100 mL

NOTE: In this study, the formulation was stored in amber plastic prescription bottles.

INSTRUCTIONS: Crush the tablets in a mortar and reduce to a fine powder. Mix the two vehicles together. Add a small amount of the vehicle to the mortar and levigate to a uniform paste. Add geometric amounts of the vehicle while mixing. Transfer to a graduate, rinse the mortar with vehicle, and transfer to graduate to qs to 100 mL. Stir well.

NOTES

GENERIC NAME	**Pyrazinamide**
DOSAGE FORM	oral suspension
MADE FROM	tablets
CONCENTRATION	100 mg/mL
STABILITY	60 days (25 °C); 45 days (4 °C)
STABILITY REFERENCE	Nahata MC, et al. Am J Health Syst Pharm 1995;52:1558-60
STORE	refrigerate (preferable) or at room temperature
LABEL	shake well before use, refrigerate

INGREDIENT	STRENGTH	QUANTITY
Pyrazinamide tablets	500 mg	20
Simple syrup, NF		qs 100 mL

NOTE: The use of methylcellulose may decrease the potential for settling, thus increasing the accuracy of measuring individual doses of pyrazinamide after storage. In this study, the formulation was stored in amber plastic prescription bottles.

INSTRUCTIONS: Crush the tablets in a mortar and triturate to a fine powder. Levigate the powder with a small portion of the vehicle to obtain a uniform paste. Add more vehicle in geometric proportions, mix thoroughly, and transfer the contents to a graduate. Rinse the mortar with small portions of the vehicle, transfer to a graduate, and qs to 100 mL.

NOTES

GENERIC NAME	**Pyrazinamide**
DOSAGE FORM	oral suspension
MADE FROM	tablets
CONCENTRATION	100 mg/mL
STABILITY	60 days (4 °C); 45 days (25 °C)
STABILITY REFERENCE	Nahata MC, et al. Am J Health Syst Pharm 1995; 52:1558-60
STORE	refrigerate (preferable) or at room temperature
LABEL	shake well before use, refrigerate

INGREDIENT	STRENGTH	QUANTITY
Pyrazinamide tablets	500 mg	20
[a]Citrucel (methylcellulose 1% solution):simple syrup, NF	1:1	qs 100 mL

[a]Prepare vehicle by mixing 2.55 g of Citrucel (containing methylcellulose 0.5 g) with small portions of distilled water to form a uniform mixture, then qs with water to 50 mL. This 50 mL is then mixed with 50 mL of simple syrup, NF.

NOTE: In this study, the formulation was stored in amber plastic prescription bottles.

INSTRUCTIONS: Crush the tablets in a mortar and triturate to a fine powder. Levigate the powder with a small portion of distilled water to obtain a uniform paste. Add vehicle in geometric proportions, mix thoroughly, and transfer the contents to a graduate. Rinse the mortar with small portions of the vehicle, transfer to a graduate, and qs to 100 mL.

NOTES

GENERIC NAME	**Pyrazinamide**
DOSAGE FORM	oral suspension
MADE FROM	tablets
CONCENTRATION	10 mg/mL
STABILITY	60 days
STABILITY REFERENCE	Allen LV, et al. Am J Health Syst Pharm 1998;55:1804-9
STORE	refrigerate (preferable) or at room temperature
LABEL	shake well before use, refrigerate

INGREDIENT	STRENGTH	QUANTITY
Pyrazinamide tablets	500 mg	3
Ora-Plus:Ora-Sweet or Ora-Plus:Ora-Sweet SF	1:1	qs 150 mL

NOTE: In this study, the formulation was stored in amber clear plastic (polyethylene terephthalate) prescription bottles.

INSTRUCTIONS: Triturate the tablets to a fine powder. Add approximately 10 mL of the vehicle and levigate to a uniform paste. Add the vehicle in geometric proportions almost to volume, mix thoroughly, and transfer to a graduate. Rinse the mortar with the vehicle, transfer to the graduate, and qs to 150 mL.

NOTES

GENERIC NAME	**Pyrazinamide**
DOSAGE FORM	oral suspension
MADE FROM	tablets
CONCENTRATION	10 mg/mL
STABILITY	60 days
STABILITY REFERENCE	Allen LV, et al. Am J Health Syst Pharm 1998; 55:1804-9
STORE	refrigerate (preferable) or at room temperature
LABEL	shake well before use, refrigerate

INGREDIENT	STRENGTH	QUANTITY
Pyrazinamide tablets	500 mg	3
Cherry syrup (cherry syrup concentrate diluted 1:4 with simple syrup, NF)		qs 150 mL

NOTE: In this study, the formulation was stored in amber clear plastic (polyethylene terephthalate) prescription bottles.

INSTRUCTIONS: Triturate the tablets to a fine powder. Add approximately 10 mL of the vehicle and levigate to a uniform paste. Add the vehicle in geometric proportions almost to volume, mix thoroughly, and transfer to a graduate. Rinse the mortar with the vehicle, transfer to the graduate, and qs to 150 mL.

NOTES

Pyridoxine Hydrochloride

GENERIC NAME	
DOSAGE FORM	oral solution
MADE FROM	injection
CONCENTRATION	1 mg/mL
STABILITY	30 days
STABILITY REFERENCE	experience
STORE	refrigerate
LABEL	refrigerate

INGREDIENT	STRENGTH	QUANTITY
Pyridoxine hydrochloride injection	100 mg/mL	1 mL
Simple syrup, NF		qs ad 100 mL

INSTRUCTIONS: Withdraw the pyridoxine solution from a vial with a syringe and add to 99 mL of syrup. Dispense in an amber glass bottle.

NOTES

GENERIC NAME	**Pyrimethamine**
DOSAGE FORM	oral suspension
MADE FROM	tablets
CONCENTRATION	2 mg/mL
STABILITY	91 days
STABILITY REFERENCE	Nahata MC, et al. Am J Health Syst Pharm 1997; 54:2714-6
STORE	refrigerate (preferable) or at room temperature
LABEL	shake well before use, refrigerate

INGREDIENT	STRENGTH	QUANTITY
Pyrimethamine tablets	25 mg	40
Simple syrup, NF: methylcellulose 1%	1:1	qs 500 mL

NOTE: In this study, the formulation was stored in amber plastic prescription bottles.

INSTRUCTIONS: Crush the tablets in a mortar and triturate to a fine powder. Levigate the powder with a small portion of the vehicle to form a uniform paste. Add more vehicle in geometric proportions, mix thoroughly, and transfer to a graduate. Rinse the mortar with vehicle repeatedly, transfer the rinsings to the graduate, and qs to 500 mL.

NOTES

GENERIC NAME	**Quinapril Hydrochloride**
DOSAGE FORM	oral suspension
MADE FROM	tablets
CONCENTRATION	1 mg/mL
STABILITY	42 days
STABILITY REFERENCE	Freed AL, et al. Int J Pharm 2005;304(1-2): 135-44
STORE	refrigerate
LABEL	shake well before use, refrigerate

INGREDIENT	STRENGTH	QUANTITY
Quinapril hydrochloride tablets	20 mg	10
KPhos neutral tablet		1
Bicitra		30 mL
Sterile Water for Irrigation		100 mL
Ora-Sweet or Ora-Sweet SF		140 mL

NOTE: In this study, the formulation was stored in amber-colored polyethylene terephthalate with screw caps. Some particles settled after 15 minutes in the formulation continuing ora-sweet, but the stability was unaffected. Each KPhos neutral tablet contains 852 mg dibasic sodium phosphate anhydrous, 155 mg monobasic potassium phosphate, and 130 mg monobasic sodium phosphate monohydrate, to yield approximately 250 mg phosphate, 298 mg sodium (13.0 mEq) and 45 mg of potassium (1.1 mEq) per tablet. Bicitra contains sodium citrate dihydrate (500 mg/5 mL) and citric acid monohydrate (334 mg/5 mL).

INSTRUCTIONS: Prepare KPhos buffer solution by dissolving one KPhos neutral tablet in 100 mL of sterile water for irrigation. Add 30 mL of this solution to a 200-mL amber-colored polyethylene terephthalate with screw cap containing ten quinapril tablets; shake for 2 minutes with screw cap on. Remove the screw cap and let the concentrate stand for 15 minutes. Shake again for an additional minute. Add 30 mL of Bicitra and shake for an additional 2 minutes. Add 140 mL of Ora-Sweet and shake to disperse the suspension.

NOTES

GENERIC NAME	**Quinapril Hydrochloride**
DOSAGE FORM	oral suspension
MADE FROM	tablets
CONCENTRATION	1 mg/mL
STABILITY	42 days
STABILITY REFERENCE	Freed AL, et al. Int J Pharm 2005;304(1-2): 135-44
STORE	refrigerate
LABEL	shake well before use, refrigerate

INGREDIENT	STRENGTH	QUANTITY
Quinapril hydrochloride tablets	20 mg	10
KPhos neutral tablet		1
Bicitra		30 mL
Sterile water for irrigation		100 mL
Simple syrup, NF		140 mL

NOTE:	In this study, the formulation was stored in amber-colored polyethylene terephthalate with screw caps. Of the three formulations, some particles settled after a few minutes. Each KPhos neutral tablet contains 852 mg dibasic sodium phosphate anhydrous, 155 mg monobasic potassium phosphate, and 130 mg monobasic sodium phosphate monohydrate, to yield approximately 250 mg phosphate, 298 mg sodium (13.0 mEq), and 45 mg of potassium (1.1 mEq) per tablet. Bicitra contains sodium citrate dihydrate (500 mg/5 mL) and citric acid monohydrate (334 mg/5 mL).
INSTRUCTIONS:	Prepare KPhos buffer solution by dissolving 1 KPhos neutral tablet in 100 mL of sterile water for irrigation. Add 30 mL of this solution to a 200-mL amber-colored polyethylene terephthalate with screw cap containing ten quinapril tablets; shake for 2 minutes with screw cap on. Remove the screw cap and let the concentrate stand for 15 minutes. Shake again for an additional minute. Add 30 mL of Bicitra and shake for an additional 2 minutes. Add 140 mL of simple syrup and shake to disperse the suspension.

NOTES

GENERIC NAME	**Quinidine**
DOSAGE FORM	oral suspension
MADE FROM	tablets
CONCENTRATION	10 mg/mL
STABILITY	60 days
STABILITY REFERENCE	Allen LV, et al. Am J Health Syst Pharm 1998;55: 1804-9
STORE	refrigerate (preferable) or at room temperature
LABEL	shake well before use, refrigerate

INGREDIENT	STRENGTH	QUANTITY
Quinidine sulfate tablets	200 mg	6
Ora-Plus:Ora-Sweet or Ora-Plus:Ora-Sweet SF	1:1 mixture	qs 120 mL

NOTE: In this study, the formulation was stored in amber clear plastic (polyethylene terephthalate) prescription bottles.

INSTRUCTIONS: Crush the tablets and triturate to a fine powder. Add approximately 15 mL of vehicle and levigate to a uniform paste. Add vehicle in geometric proportions almost to volume, mix thoroughly, and transfer to a graduate. Rinse the mortar with vehicle, add to the graduate, and qs to 120 mL.

NOTES

GENERIC NAME	**Quinidine**
DOSAGE FORM	oral suspension
MADE FROM	tablets
CONCENTRATION	10 mg/mL
STABILITY	60 days
STABILITY REFERENCE	Allen LV, et al. Am J Health Syst Pharm 1998; 55:1804-9
STORE	refrigerate (preferable) or at room temperature
LABEL	shake well before use, refrigerate

INGREDIENT	STRENGTH	QUANTITY
Quinidine sulfate tablets	200 mg	6
Cherry syrup (cherry syrup concentrate diluted 1:4 with simple syrup, NF)		qs 120 mL

NOTE: In this study, the formulation was stored in amber clear plastic (polyethylene terephthalate) prescription bottles.

INSTRUCTIONS: Crush the tablets and triturate to a fine powder. Add approximately 15 mL of vehicle and levigate to a uniform paste. Add vehicle in geometric proportions almost to volume, mix thoroughly, and transfer to a graduate. Rinse the mortar with vehicle, add to the graduate, and qs to 120 mL.

NOTES

GENERIC NAME	**Ranitidine**
DOSAGE FORM	injection
MADE FROM	injection
CONCENTRATION	2.5 mg/mL
STABILITY	91 days
STABILITY REFERENCE	Nahata MC, et al. Am J Health Syst Pharm 1996;53:1588-90
STORE	refrigerate
LABEL	refrigerate

INGREDIENT	STRENGTH	QUANTITY
Ranitidine injection	25 mg/mL	1 mL
Bacteriostatic water for injection		9 mL

NOTE: In this study, the formulation was stored in glass vials and plastic syringes.

INSTRUCTIONS: Mix the ingredients in an empty sterile vial using aseptic technique.

NOTES

GENERIC NAME	**Ranitidine**
DOSAGE FORM	oral suspension
MADE FROM	tablets
CONCENTRATION	15 mg/mL
STABILITY	7 days
STABILITY REFERENCE	Karnes HT, et al. Am J Hosp Pharm 1989;46: 304-7
STORE	room temperature
LABEL	shake well before use

INGREDIENT	STRENGTH	QUANTITY
Ranitidine hydrochloride tablets	150 mg	10
Distilled water		50 ml
Simple syrup, NF		qs 100 mL

NOTE: In this study, the formulation was stored in amber bottles. Commercially available as a syrup, 15 mg/mL.

INSTRUCTIONS: Crush the tablets and triturate into a fine powder. Levigate with a small amount of distilled water into a uniform paste. Add the remaining water in geometric proportions, mix thoroughly, and transfer to a graduate. Rinse the mortar with simple syrup, transfer to the graduate, and qs to 100 mL. Sonicate the suspension for 15 minutes to obtain a homogenous suspension.

NOTES

GENERIC NAME	**Rifabutin**
DOSAGE FORM	oral suspension
MADE FROM	capsules
CONCENTRATION	20 mg/mL
STABILITY	84 days (4 °C, 25 °C, 30 °C)
STABILITY REFERENCE	Haslam JL, et al. Am J Health Syst Pharm 1999;56:333-6
STORE	refrigerate (preferable) or at room temperature
LABEL	shake well before use, refrigerate

INGREDIENT	STRENGTH	QUANTITY
Rifabutin capsules	150 mg	8
Ora-Plus:Ora-Sweet	1:1 mixture	qs 60 mL

NOTE: In this study, the formulation was stored in amber polyethylene terephthalate glycol prescription ovals.

INSTRUCTIONS: Empty the contents of the capsules into a mortar and triturate to a fine powder. Add approximately 20 mL of the vehicle and levigate to a uniform paste. Add vehicle in geometric proportions almost to volume, mix thoroughly, and transfer to a graduate. Rinse the mortar with vehicle, add to the graduate, and qs to 60 mL.

NOTES

GENERIC NAME	**Rifabutin**
DOSAGE FORM	oral suspension
MADE FROM	capsules
CONCENTRATION	20 mg/mL
STABILITY	84 days (4 °C, 25 °C, 30 °C); 56 days (40 °C)
STABILITY REFERENCE	Haslam JL, et al. Am J Health Syst Pharm 1999; 56:333-6
STORE	refrigerate (preferable) or at room temperature
LABEL	shake well before use, refrigerate

INGREDIENT	STRENGTH	QUANTITY
Rifabutin capsules	150 mg	8
Cherry syrup, USP		qs 60 mL

NOTE: In this study, the formulation was stored in amber plastic (polyethylene terephthalate) glycol prescription ovals.

INSTRUCTIONS: Empty the contents of the capsules into a mortar and triturate to a fine powder. Add approximately 20 mL of the vehicle and levigate to a uniform paste. Add vehicle in geometric proportions almost to volume, mix thoroughly, and transfer to a graduate. Rinse the mortar with vehicle, add to the graduate, and qs to 60 mL.

NOTES

GENERIC NAME	**Rifampin**
DOSAGE FORM	oral suspension
MADE FROM	powder
CONCENTRATION	10 mg/mL
STABILITY	30 days
STABILITY REFERENCE	Rifampin oral suspension. United States Pharmacopeia XXIII/National Formulary 18. Supplement 9. November 1998:4601
STORE	room temperature, in tight, light-resistant glass or plastic prescription bottle
LABEL	shake well before use

INGREDIENT	STRENGTH	QUANTITY
Rifampin powder		1.2 g
Rifampin capsules	300 mg	4
Simple syrup, NF		qs 120 mL

INSTRUCTIONS: Transfer rifampin powder or the contents of rifampin capsules into a mortar. Triturate the contents to obtain a fine powder. Add approximately 2 mL of syrup and levigate until a smooth paste is formed. Add syrup in geometric proportions until approximately 80 mL has been added. Transfer the suspension to a graduate and qs to 120 mL with syrup. Mix well to produce a suspension.

NOTES

Copyright © 2011 Harvey Whitney Books

GENERIC NAME	**Rifampin**
DOSAGE FORM	oral suspension
MADE FROM	capsules
CONCENTRATION	25 mg/mL
STABILITY	28 days
STABILITY REFERENCE	Allen LV, et al. Am J Health Syst Pharm 1998; 55:1804-9
STORE	refrigerate (preferable) or at room temperature
LABEL	shake well before use, refrigerate

INGREDIENT	STRENGTH	QUANTITY
Rifampin capsules	300 mg	10
Ora-Plus:Ora-Sweet	1:1	
or Ora-Plus:Ora-Sweet SF		qs 120 mL

NOTE: In this study, the formulation was stored in amber clear plastic (polyethylene terephthalate) prescription ovals.

INSTRUCTIONS: Empty the contents of the capsules into a mortar. Triturate to a fine powder until thoroughly mixed. Add approximately 20 mL of the vehicle and levigate to a uniform paste. Add vehicle in geometric proportions almost to volume, mix thoroughly, and transfer to a graduate. Rinse the mortar with vehicle, add to the graduate, and qs to 120 mL.

NOTES

GENERIC NAME	**Rifampin**
DOSAGE FORM	oral suspension
MADE FROM	capsules
CONCENTRATION	25 mg/mL
STABILITY	28 days
STABILITY REFERENCE	Allen LV, et al. Am J Health Syst Pharm 1998;55:1804-9
STORE	refrigerate (preferable) or at room temperature
LABEL	shake well before use, refrigerate

INGREDIENT	STRENGTH	QUANTITY
Rifampin capsules	300 mg	10
Cherry syrup (cherry syrup concentrate diluted 1:4 with simple syrup, NF)		qs 120 mL

NOTE:	In this study, the formulation was stored in amber clear plastic (polyethylene terephthalate) prescription ovals.
INSTRUCTIONS:	Empty the contents of the capsules into a mortar. Triturate to a fine powder until thoroughly mixed. Add approximately 20 mL of the vehicle and levigate to a uniform paste. Add vehicle in geometric proportions almost to volume, mix thoroughly, and transfer to a graduate. Rinse the mortar with vehicle, add to the graduate, and qs to 120 mL.

NOTES

GENERIC NAME	**Rifampin**
DOSAGE FORM	oral suspension
MADE FROM	capsules
CONCENTRATION	10 mg/mL
STABILITY	42 days
STABILITY REFERENCE	Nahata MC, et al. J Clin Pharm Ther 1994;19: 263-5
STORE	room temperature
LABEL	shake well before use

INGREDIENT	STRENGTH	QUANTITY
Rifampin capsules	300 mg	4
Simple syrup, NF		qs 120 mL

NOTE: In this study, the formulation was stored in plastic prescription bottles.

INSTRUCTIONS: Empty the contents of the capsules into a mortar. Triturate to a fine powder and mix uniformly. Add 20 mL of the vehicle and levigate into a smooth paste. Add vehicle in geometric proportions almost to volume, mix thoroughly, and transfer the contents to a graduate. Rinse the mortar with the vehicle, add to the graduate, and qs to 120 mL.

NOTES

GENERIC NAME	**Rifampin**
DOSAGE FORM	oral suspension
MADE FROM	injection
CONCENTRATION	10 mg/mL
STABILITY	56 days
STABILITY REFERENCE	Nahata MC, et al. J Clin Pharm Ther 1994;19:263-5
STORE	room temperature
LABEL	shake well before use

INGREDIENT	STRENGTH	QUANTITY
Rifampin powder for injection	600 mg	2 vials
Simple syrup, NF		qs 120 mL

NOTE: In this study, the formulation was stored in plastic prescription bottles.

INSTRUCTIONS: Reconstitute each vial with 10 mL of sterile water for injection. Empty the contents of the vials into a mortar after reconstitution. Add the vehicle in geometric proportions, mix thoroughly, and transfer the contents to a graduate. Rinse the mortar with the vehicle, add to the graduate, and qs to 120 mL.

NOTES

GENERIC NAME	**Rifaximin**
DOSAGE FORM	oral suspension
MADE FROM	tablets
CONCENTRATION	20 mg/mL
STABILITY	60 days
STABILITY REFERENCE	Cober MP, et. al. Am J Health Syst Pharm 2010; 67:287-9
STORE	room temperature
LABEL	shake well before use, protect from light

INGREDIENT	STRENGTH	QUANTITY
Rifaximin tablets	200 mg	6
Ora-Plus		30 mL
Ora-Sweet		30 mL

NOTE: In this study, the formulation was stored in amber-colored child-resistant prescription bottles.

INSTRUCTIONS: Triturate six tablets into a fine powder in a glass mortar. Mix equal quantities of Ora-Plus and Ora-Sweet in geometric proportions with constant stirring to produce 60 mL. Using 30 mL of this mixture, levigate the powder into a smooth suspension, adding the vehicle in geometric proportions. Transfer the suspension to a 2-oz child-resistant amber prescription bottle. Rinse the mortar with sufficient vehicle to bring the final volume in the bottle to 60 mL.

NOTES

GENERIC NAME	**Rufinamide**
DOSAGE FORM	oral suspension
MADE FROM	tablets
CONCENTRATION	40 mg/mL
STABILITY	90 days
STABILITY REFERENCE	Hutchinson DJ, et al. Ann Pharmacother 2010; 44:462-5
STORE	room temperature
LABEL	shake well before use, protect from light

INGREDIENT	STRENGTH	QUANTITY
Rufinamide tablets	400 mg	12
Ora-Plus		60 mL
Ora-Sweet or Ora-Sweet SF		60 mL

NOTE: In this study, the formulation was stored in amber-colored prescription bottles.

INSTRUCTIONS: Triturate twelve tablets into a fine powder in a glass mortar. Mix equal quantities of Ora-Plus and Ora-Sweet in geometric proportions with constant stirring to produce 120 mL. Using 30 mL of this mixture, levigate the powder into a smooth suspension, adding the vehicle in geometric proportions. Transfer the suspension to a graduate. Rinse the mortar with sufficient vehicle to bring the final volume in the bottle to 120 mL.

NOTES

GENERIC NAME	**Shohl's Solution**
DOSAGE FORM	oral solution
MADE FROM	powder
CONCENTRATION	1 mEq sodium/mL
STABILITY	30 days
STABILITY REFERENCE	experience
STORE	room temperature

INGREDIENT	STRENGTH	QUANTITY
Citric acid		140 g
Sodium citrate		90 g
Purified water, USP		qs ad 1000 g

INSTRUCTIONS: Dissolve the two citrates in water and qs to volume.

NOTES

GENERIC NAME	**Sildenafil**
DOSAGE FORM	oral suspension
MADE FROM	tablets
CONCENTRATION	2.5 mg/mL
STABILITY	91 days
STABILITY REFERENCE	Nahata MC, et al. Presented at: American Society of Health-System Pharmacists Midyear Clinical Meeting, December 9, 2003 (poster)
STORE	refrigerate (preferable) or room temperature
LABEL	refrigerate, shake well before use

INGREDIENT	STRENGTH	QUANTITY
Sildenafil tablets (Revatio)	20 mg	15
Simple syrup, NF: 1% methylcellulose suspension	1:7	qs 120 mL

NOTE:	This formulation was stored in amber plastic prescription bottles.
INSTRUCTIONS:	Mix simple syrup and 1% methylcellulose suspension together thoroughly in a glass mortar, in geometric proportions, to prepare the vehicle. Triturate the tablets into a fine powder and levigate with small proportion of the vehicle into a smooth suspension. Add vehicle in geometric proportions with constant mixing. Transfer to a graduate. Rinse the mortar with sufficient vehicle and transfer to graduate to make up the final volume.

NOTES

GENERIC NAME	**Sildenafil**
DOSAGE FORM	oral suspension
MADE FROM	tablets
CONCENTRATION	2.5 mg/mL
STABILITY	91 days
STABILITY REFERENCE	Nahata MC, et al. Presented at: American Society of Health-System Pharmacists Midyear Clinical Meeting, December 2003
STORE	refrigerate (preferable) or room temperature
LABEL	refrigerate, shake well before use

INGREDIENT	STRENGTH	QUANTITY
Sildenafil tablets (Revatio)	20 mg	15
Ora-Plus:Ora-Sweet	1:1	qs 120 mL

NOTE: This formulation was stored in amber plastic prescription bottles.

INSTRUCTIONS: Mix Ora-Plus and Ora-Sweet together thoroughly in a glass mortar, in geometric proportions, to prepare the vehicle. Triturate the tablets into a fine powder and levigate with small proportion of the vehicle into a smooth suspension. Add vehicle in geometric proportions, with constant mixing. Transfer to a graduate. Rinse the mortar with sufficient vehicle and transfer to graduate to make up the final volume.

NOTES

GENERIC NAME	**Sildenafil**
DOSAGE FORM	oral suspension
MADE FROM	tablets
CONCENTRATION	2.5 mg/mL
STABILITY	91 days
STABILITY REFERENCE	Nahata MC, et al. Am J Health Syst Pharm 2006;63:254-7
STORE	refrigerate (preferable) or room temperature
LABEL	refrigerate, shake well before use

INGREDIENT	STRENGTH	QUANTITY
Sildenafil tablets (Viagra)	25 mg	30
Simple syrup, NF: 1% methylcellulose suspension	1:1	qs 300 mL

NOTE: This formulation was stored in amber plastic prescription bottles.

INSTRUCTIONS: Mix simple syrup and 1% methylcellulose suspension thoroughly, using a glass mortar and pestle, in geometric proportions, to prepare the vehicle. Triturate the tablets into a fine powder and levigate with small proportions of the vehicle into a smooth suspension. Add vehicle in geometric proportions with constant mixing. Transfer to a graduate. Rinse the mortar with sufficient vehicle and transfer to graduate to make up the final volume.

NOTES

GENERIC NAME	**Sildenafil**
DOSAGE FORM	oral suspension
MADE FROM	tablets
CONCENTRATION	2.5 mg/mL
STABILITY	91 days
STABILITY REFERENCE	Nahata MC, et al. Am J Health Syst Pharm. 2006;63:254-7
STORE	refrigerate (preferable) or room temperature
LABEL	refrigerate, shake well before use

INGREDIENT	STRENGTH	QUANTITY
Sildenafil tablets (Viagra)	25 mg	30
Ora-Plus:Ora-Sweet	1:1	qs 300 mL

NOTE: This formulation was stored in amber plastic prescription bottles.

INSTRUCTIONS: Mix Ora-Plus and Ora-Sweet together thoroughly in a glass mortar, in geometric proportions, to prepare the vehicle. Triturate the tablets into a fine powder and levigate with small proportion of the vehicle into a smooth suspension. Add vehicle in geometric proportions with constant mixing. Transfer to a graduate. Rinse the mortar with sufficient vehicle and transfer to graduate to make up the final volume.

NOTES

GENERIC NAME	**Sodium Bicarbonate**
DOSAGE FORM	oral solution
MADE FROM	powder
CONCENTRATION	1 mEq/mL
STABILITY	30 days
STABILITY REFERENCE	Reynolds JEF, ed. Martindale: the extra pharmacopoeia. 29th ed. London: Pharmaceutical Press, 1989:1027
STORE	room temperature in amber glass bottles

INGREDIENT	STRENGTH	QUANTITY
Sodium bicarbonate powder		84 g
Purified water, USP		qs ad 1000 mL

INSTRUCTIONS: Dissolve the powder in water and package immediately.

NOTES

GENERIC NAME	**Sodium Hypochlorite**
DOSAGE FORM	topical solution
MADE FROM	powder
CONCENTRATION	0.025%
STABILITY	7 days
STABILITY REFERENCE	ASHP technical assistance bulletin on pharmacy-prepared ophthalmic products. Am J Hosp Pharm 1993;50:1462-3
STORE	room temperature, in tight, light-resistant plastic containers
LABEL	for external use only

INGREDIENT	STRENGTH	QUANTITY
Sodium hypochlorite solution	(5.25% w/v)	5 mL
Monobasic sodium phosphate monohydrate		1.02 g
Dibasic sodium phosphate anhydrous		17.61 g
Purified water		qs 1000 mL

INSTRUCTIONS: Dissolve the dibasic sodium phosphate anhydrous and the monobasic sodium phosphate monohydrate in approximately 500 mL of purified water. Add the sodium hypochlorite solution and purified water, qs to 1000 mL, and mix.

NOTES

GENERIC NAME	**Sodium Hypochlorite (Dakin's 0.125% solution)**
DOSAGE FORM	topical solution
MADE FROM	solution
CONCENTRATION	0.125%
STABILITY	30 days protected from light; 24 hours if not protected from light
STABILITY REFERENCE	experience
STORE	room temperature
LABEL	protect from light

INGREDIENT	STRENGTH	QUANTITY
Sodium hypochlorite solution	5.25%	25 mL
Distilled water		qs 1000 mL

NOTE: In this study, the formulation was stored in amber glass bottles.

INSTRUCTIONS: Measure bleach into a graduate. Add distilled water in geometric proportions with constant stirring to make up the final volume.

NOTES

GENERIC NAME	**Sodium Hypochlorite**
DOSAGE FORM	topical solution
MADE FROM	solution
CONCENTRATION	1:8 (0.125%)
STABILITY	23 months
STABILITY REFERENCE	Fabian TM, et al. Am J Hosp Pharm 1982;39: 1016-7
STORE	protect from light

INGREDIENT	STRENGTH	QUANTITY
Sodium hypochlorite solution	1%	25 mL
Distilled water		qs 200 mL

NOTE: In this study, the formulation was stored in amber glass bottles.

INSTRUCTIONS: Measure bleach into a graduate. Add distilled water in geometric proportions, with constant stirring, to make up the final volume.

NOTES

GENERIC NAME	**Sodium Hypochlorite**
DOSAGE FORM	topical solution
MADE FROM	solution
CONCENTRATION	1:12 (0.083%)
STABILITY	23 months
STABILITY REFERENCE	Fabian TM, et al. Am J Hosp Pharm 1982;39: 1016-7
STORE	protect from light

INGREDIENT	STRENGTH	QUANTITY
Sodium hypochlorite solution	1%	25 mL
Distilled water		qs 300 mL

NOTE: In this study, the formulation was stored in amber glass bottles.

INSTRUCTIONS: Measure bleach into a graduate. Add distilled water in geometric proportions, with constant stirring, to make up the final volume.

NOTES

GENERIC NAME	**Sodium Hypochlorite**
DOSAGE FORM	topical solution
MADE FROM	solution
CONCENTRATION	1:20 (0.05%)
STABILITY	23 months
STABILITY REFERENCE	Fabian TM, et al. Am J Hosp Pharm 1982;39: 1016-7
STORE	protect from light

INGREDIENT	STRENGTH	QUANTITY
Sodium hypochlorite solution	1%	25 mL
Distilled water		qs 500 mL

NOTE: In this study, the formulation was stored in amber glass bottles.

INSTRUCTIONS: Measure bleach into a graduate. Add distilled water in geometric proportions, with constant stirring, to make up the final volume.

NOTES

GENERIC NAME	**Sodium Phenylbutyrate**
DOSAGE FORM	oral suspension
MADE FROM	powder
CONCENTRATION	200 mg/mL
STABILITY	90 days
STABILITY REFERENCE	Caruthers RL, et al. Am J Health Syst Pharm 2007;64:1513-5
STORE	room temperature
LABEL	shake well before use, protect from light

INGREDIENT	STRENGTH	QUANTITY
Sodium phenylbutyrate USP		12 g
Ora-Plus		30 mL
Ora-Sweet		30 mL

NOTE: In this study, the formulation was stored in amber-colored child-resistant plastic bottles.

INSTRUCTIONS: Triturate sodium phenylbutyrate USP into a fine powder in a glass mortar. Mix equal quantities of Ora-Plus and Ora-Sweet in geometric proportions with constant stirring to produce 60 mL. Using 30 mL of this mixture, levigate the powder into a smooth suspension, adding the vehicle in geometric proportions. Transfer the suspension to a 2-oz child-resistant amber plastic bottle. Rinse the mortar with sufficient vehicle and transfer into the bottle to bring the final volume to 60 mL.

NOTES

GENERIC NAME	**Sodium Phenylbutyrate**
DOSAGE FORM	oral suspension
MADE FROM	powder
CONCENTRATION	200 mg/mL
STABILITY	90 days
STABILITY REFERENCE	Caruthers RL, et al. Am J Health Syst Pharm 2007;64:1513-5
STORE	room temperature
LABEL	shake well before use, protect from light

INGREDIENT	STRENGTH	QUANTITY
Sodium pheynlbutyrate, USP		12 g
Ora-Plus		30 mL
Ora-Sweet SF		30 mL

NOTE: In this study, the formulation was stored in amber-colored child-resistant plastic bottles.

INSTRUCTIONS: Triturate sodium phenylbutyrate, USP, into a fine powder in a glass mortar. Mix equal quantities of Ora-Plus and Ora-Sweet SF in geometric proportions with constant stirring to produce 60 mL. Using 30 mL of this mixture, levigate the powder into a smooth suspension, adding the vehicle in geometric proportions. Transfer the suspension to a 2-oz child-resistant amber plastic bottle. Rinse the mortar with sufficient vehicle and transfer into the bottle to bring the final volume to 60 mL.

NOTES

GENERIC NAME	**Sotalol**
DOSAGE FORM	oral suspension
MADE FROM	tablets
CONCENTRATION	5 mg/mL
STABILITY	56 days
STABILITY REFERENCE	Dupuis LL, et al. Can J Hosp Pharm 1988;41:121-3
STORE	refrigerate
LABEL	shake well before use, refrigerate

INGREDIENT	STRENGTH	QUANTITY
Sotalol hydrochloride tablets	160 mg	5
Simple syrup, NF		48 mL
[a]Methylcellulose gel	1%	112 mL

[a]Sodium benzoate 6 g, methylcellulose cps 1500 30 g, water for irrigation qs 3000 mL. Measure 600 mL of boiling water for irrigation into blender. Add sodium benzoate and mix to dissolve. With blender on, add methylcellulose powder to sodium benzoate solution. Add 2400 mL of ice-cold water for irrigation quickly to the mixture and mix for an additional 10 minutes. Transfer to amber glass bottles. Refrigerate for a minimum of 4 hours before use, after which the gel may be stored at room temperature. Expiration: 6 months.

NOTE: In this study, the formulation was stored in air-tight glass vials stoppered with rubber tops and sealed with aluminum caps.

INSTRUCTIONS: Mix simple syrup and methylcellulose gel in geometric proportions in a blender. Store at room temperature and protect from light for at least 4 hours before use. Crush the tablets and triturate into a fine powder in a mortar. Levigate the powder with a small amount of vehicle into a smooth paste. Add vehicle in geometric proportions almost to volume, mix thoroughly, and transfer to a graduate. Rinse the mortar with vehicle, add to the graduate, and qs to 160 mL.

NOTES

GENERIC NAME	**Sotalol**
DOSAGE FORM	oral suspension
MADE FROM	tablets
CONCENTRATION	5 mg/mL
STABILITY	91 days
STABILITY REFERENCE	Nahata MC, et al. Presented at: American Society of Health-System Pharmacists Midyear Clinical Meeting, Las Vegas, December 3–7, 2000 (poster)
STORE	refrigerate (preferable) or at room temperature
LABEL	shake well before use, refrigerate

INGREDIENT	STRENGTH	QUANTITY
Sotalol hydrochloride tablets	120 mg	5
Methylcellulose	1%	12 mL
Simple syrup, NF		qs 120 mL

NOTE: In this study, the formulation was stored in plastic prescription bottles.

INSTRUCTIONS: Crush the tablets and triturate to mix well. Levigate the powder with methylcellulose gel to obtain a uniform paste. Add syrup in geometric proportions, mix well, and transfer to a graduate. Rinse the mortar with syrup, transfer to graduate, and qs to 120 mL.

NOTES

GENERIC NAME	**Sotalol**
DOSAGE FORM	oral suspension
MADE FROM	tablets
CONCENTRATION	5 mg/mL
STABILITY	91 days
STABILITY REFERENCE	Nahata MC, et al. Presented at: American Society of Health-System Pharmacists Midyear Clinical Meeting, Las Vegas, December 3–7, 2000 (poster)
STORE	refrigerate (preferable) or at room temperature
LABEL	shake well before use, refrigerate

INGREDIENT	STRENGTH	QUANTITY
Sotalol hydrochloride tablets	120 mg	5
Ora-Plus:Ora-Sweet	1:1	qs 120 mL

NOTE: In this study, the formulation was stored in plastic prescription bottles.

INSTRUCTIONS: Crush the tablets and triturate to mix well. Levigate the powder with vehicle to obtain a uniform paste. Add vehicle in geometric proportions, mix well, and transfer to a graduate. Rinse the mortar with vehicle, transfer to graduate, and qs to 120 mL.

NOTES

GENERIC NAME	**Spironolactone**
DOSAGE FORM	oral suspension
MADE FROM	tablets
CONCENTRATION	25 mg/mL
STABILITY	60 days
STABILITY REFERENCE	Allen LV Jr, et al. Am J Health Syst Pharm 1996; 53:2073-8
STORE	refrigerate (preferable) or at room temperature
LABEL	shake well before use, refrigerate

INGREDIENT	STRENGTH	QUANTITY
Spironolactone tablets	25 mg	120
Ora-Plus:Ora-Sweet or Ora-Plus:Ora-Sweet SF	1:1	qs 120 mL

NOTE: In this study, the formulation was stored in amber clear plastic (polyethylene terephthalate) prescription ovals.

INSTRUCTIONS: Crush the tablets and triturate to a fine powder including the tablet coating. Add approximately 20 mL of vehicle and levigate to a uniform paste. Add vehicle in geometric proportions almost to volume, mix thoroughly, and transfer to a graduate. Rinse the mortar with vehicle, add to the graduate, and qs to 120 mL.

NOTES

GENERIC NAME	**Spironolactone**
DOSAGE FORM	oral suspension
MADE FROM	tablets
CONCENTRATION	25 mg/mL
STABILITY	60 days
STABILITY REFERENCE	Allen LV Jr, et al. Am J Health Syst Pharm 1996;53:2073-8
STORE	refrigerate (preferable) or at room temperature
LABEL	shake well before use, refrigerate

INGREDIENT	STRENGTH	QUANTITY
Spironolactone tablets	25 mg	120
Cherry syrup (cherry syrup concentrate diluted 1:4 with simple syrup, NF)		qs 120 mL

NOTE: In this study, the formulation was stored in amber clear plastic (polyethylene terephthalate) prescription ovals.

INSTRUCTIONS: Crush the tablets and triturate to a fine powder including the tablet coating. Add approximately 40 mL of vehicle and levigate to a uniform paste. Add vehicle in geometric proportions almost to volume, mix thoroughly, and transfer to a graduate. Rinse the mortar with vehicle, add to the graduate, and qs to 120 mL.

NOTES

Copyright © 2011 Harvey Whitney Books

GENERIC NAME	**Spironolactone**
DOSAGE FORM	oral suspension
MADE FROM	tablets
CONCENTRATION	1 mg/mL
STABILITY	91 days
STABILITY REFERENCE	Nahata MC, et al. Ann Pharmacother 1993;27: 1198-9
STORE	refrigerate (preferable) or at room temperature
LABEL	shake well before use, refrigerate

INGREDIENT	STRENGTH	QUANTITY
Spironolactone tablets	25 mg	10
Carboxymethylcellulose sodium	1.5%	50 mL
Simple syrup, NF		100 mL
Purified water, USP		qs ad 250 mL

INSTRUCTIONS: Put the tablets and a small amount of water in a blender and allow to soak for 5 minutes. Add carboxymethylcellulose and syrup to the blender and mix. Transfer to a graduate and qs to volume with water.

NOTES

GENERIC NAME	**Spironolactone**
DOSAGE FORM	oral suspension
MADE FROM	tablets
CONCENTRATION	10 mg/mL
STABILITY	28 days
STABILITY REFERENCE	Mathur LK, et al. Am J Hosp Pharm 1989;46:2040-2
STORE	refrigerate (preferable) or at room temperature
LABEL	shake well before use, refrigerate

INGREDIENT	STRENGTH	QUANTITY
Spironolactone tablets	100 mg	10
Purified water, USP		5 mL
Cherry syrup, USP		qs 100 mL

NOTE: In this study, the formulation was stored in type III glass prescription bottles.

INSTRUCTIONS: Crush the tablets and triturate to a fine powder including the tablet coating. Add water and levigate into a smooth paste. Add cherry syrup in geometric proportions, mix thoroughly, and transfer to a graduate. Rinse the mortar with cherry syrup, add to the graduate, and qs to 100 mL.

NOTES

GENERIC NAME	**Spironolactone/ Hydrochlorothiazide**
DOSAGE FORM	oral suspension
MADE FROM	tablets
CONCENTRATION	5 mg/mL / 5 mg/mL (hydrochlorothiazide) (spirinolactone)
STABILITY	60 days
STABILITY REFERENCE	Allen LV Jr, et al. Am J Health Syst Pharm 1996; 53:2304-8
STORE	refrigerate (preferable) or at room temperature
LABEL	shake well before use, refrigerate

INGREDIENT	STRENGTH	QUANTITY
Spironolactone/ hydrochlorothiazide tablets	25 mg/25 mg	24
Ora-Plus:Ora-Sweet or Ora-Sweet SF	1:1	qs 120 mL

NOTE: In this study, the formulation was stored in amber clear plastic (polyethylene terephthalate) prescription ovals.

INSTRUCTIONS: Crush the tablets and triturate to a fine powder. Add approximately 25 mL of vehicle and levigate to a uniform paste. Add vehicle in geometric proportions almost to volume, mix thoroughly, and transfer to a graduate. Rinse the mortar with vehicle, add to the graduate, and qs to 120 mL.

NOTES

GENERIC NAME	# Spironolactone/ Hydrochlorothiazide
DOSAGE FORM	oral suspension
MADE FROM	tablets
CONCENTRATION	5 mg/mL (spirinolactone) / 5 mg/ml (hydrochlorothiazide)
STABILITY	60 days
STABILITY REFERENCE	Allen LV Jr, et al. Am J Health Syst Pharm 1996;53:2304-8
STORE	refrigerate (preferable) or at room temperature
LABEL	shake well before use

INGREDIENT	STRENGTH	QUANTITY
Spironolactone/ hydrochlorothiazide tablets	25 mg/25 mg	24
Cherry syrup (cherry syrup concentrate diluted 1:4 with simple syrup, NF)		qs 120 mL

NOTE: In this study, the formulation was stored in amber clear plastic (polyethylene terephthalate) prescription ovals.

INSTRUCTIONS: Crush the tablets and triturate to a fine powder. Add approximately 25 mL of vehicle and levigate to a uniform paste. Add vehicle in geometric proportions almost to volume, mix thoroughly, and transfer to a graduate. Rinse the mortar with vehicle, add to the graduate, and qs to 120 mL.

NOTES

GENERIC NAME	**Sucralfate**
DOSAGE FORM	oral suspension
MADE FROM	tablets
CONCENTRATION	1000 mg/15 mL (66.67 mg/mL)
STABILITY	14 days
STABILITY REFERENCE	Ferraro JM. Drug Intell Clin Pharm 1985;19:480
STORE	refrigerate
LABEL	shake well before use, refrigerate

INGREDIENT	STRENGTH	QUANTITY
Sucralfate tablets	1 g	8
Sorbitol solution	70%	40 mL
Flavor packets (Vari Flavors, Ross Laboratories, Columbus, OH)		2 packets
Sterile water for injection		qs 120 mL

NOTE: Stability-indicating analytical methods not used.

INSTRUCTIONS: Crush the tablets in a glass mortar. Add approximately 20 mL of water and levigate to form a smooth paste. Add approximately 20 mL of additional water and make a smooth slurry. Add the sorbitol solution and mix well. Dissolve the flavor packets in approximately 10 mL of water in a separate flask, add this solution to the mortar, and mix well. Transfer the suspension to a graduate. Rinse the mortar repeatedly with water, add to the graduate, and qs to 120 mL. Mix well.

NOTES

GENERIC NAME	**Sumatriptan**
DOSAGE FORM	oral suspension
MADE FROM	tablets
CONCENTRATION	5 mg/mL
STABILITY	21 days
STABILITY REFERENCE	Fish DN, et al. Am J Health Syst Pharm 1997;54:1619-22
STORE	refrigerate
LABEL	shake well before use, refrigerate

INGREDIENT	STRENGTH	QUANTITY
Sumatriptan tablets	100 mg	9
Ora-Plus		90 mL
Ora-Sweet		qs 180 mL

NOTE: In this study, the formulation was stored in amber glass bottles.

INSTRUCTIONS: Crush the tablets in a mortar and reduce to a fine powder. Add Ora-Plus 40 mL in small amounts and levigate to a uniform paste. Add an additional 50 mL of Ora-Plus in geometric proportions, mix well, and transfer to a graduate. Rinse the mortar with small amounts of Ora-Sweet, transfer to graduate, and qs to 180 mL. Stir well.

NOTES

GENERIC NAME	**Sumatriptan**
DOSAGE FORM	oral suspension
MADE FROM	tablets
CONCENTRATION	5 mg/mL
STABILITY	14 days
STABILITY REFERENCE	Fish DN, et al. Am J Health Syst Pharm 1997; 54:1619-22
STORE	refrigerate
LABEL	shake well before use, refrigerate

INGREDIENT	STRENGTH	QUANTITY
Sumatriptan tablets	100 mg	9
Ora-Plus		90 mL
Ora-Sweet SF		qs 180 mL

NOTE: In this study, the formulation was stored in amber glass bottles.

INSTRUCTIONS: Crush the tablets in a mortar and reduce to a fine powder. Add Ora-Plus 40 mL in small amounts and levigate to a uniform paste. Add an additional 50 mL of Ora-Plus in geometric proportions, mix well, and transfer to a graduate. Rinse the mortar with small amounts of Ora-Sweet SF, transfer to graduate, and qs to 180 mL. Stir well.

NOTES

GENERIC NAME	**Sunitinib**
DOSAGE FORM	oral suspension
MADE FROM	capsules
CONCENTRATION	10 mg/mL
STABILITY	60 days
STABILITY REFERENCE	Navid F, et al. Ann Pharmacother 2008 Jul;42: 962-6
STORE	refrigerate (preferable) or room temperature
LABEL	refrigerate, shake well before use

INGREDIENT	STRENGTH	QUANTITY
Sunitinib capsules	50 mg	24
Ora-Plus:Ora-Sweet	1:1	qs 120 mL

NOTE: In this study, the formulation was stored in amber polyethylene terephthalate prescription bottles with child-resistant caps.

INSTRUCTIONS: Mix Ora-Plus and Ora-Sweet in equal proportions geometrically and prepare 120 mL of the vehicle. Open the capsules and triturate the contents into a fine powder in a glass mortar. Add small quantities of the vehicle and levigate the powder into a smooth suspension. Transfer the suspension to a graduate, rinse the mortar with small quantities of the vehicle, and transfer to the graduate to make up the final volume. Stir well.

NOTES

GENERIC NAME	**Tacrolimus**
DOSAGE FORM	oral suspension
MADE FROM	capsules
CONCENTRATION	0.5 mg/mL
STABILITY	56 days
STABILITY REFERENCE	Jacobson PA, et al. Am J Health Syst Pharm 1997;54:178-80
STORE	room temperature
LABEL	shake well before use

INGREDIENT	STRENGTH	QUANTITY
Tacrolimus capsules	5 mg	6
Ora-Plus:Simple syrup, NF	1:1	qs 60 mL

NOTE: In this study, the formulation was stored in amber glass and plastic prescription bottles.

INSTRUCTIONS: Protect hands with latex gloves. Empty the capsules into a mortar and reduce to a fine powder. Gradually mix small amounts of Ora-Plus and simple syrup in gemetric proportions to form the vehicle. Add small amount of the vehicle to the mortar and levigate into a smooth paste. Add additional vehicle to the mortar in geometric proportions almost to volume. Transfer the suspension to a graduste, rinse the mortar with the vehicle and add to graduate to qs to volume.

NOTES

Terbinafine Hydrochloride

GENERIC NAME	Terbinafine Hydrochloride
DOSAGE FORM	oral suspension
MADE FROM	tablets
CONCENTRATION	25 mg/mL
STABILITY	42 days
STABILITY REFERENCE	Abdel-Rahman SM, et al. Am J Health Syst Pharm 1999;56:243-5
STORE	refrigerate (preferable) or at room temperature
LABEL	shake well before use, refrigerate

INGREDIENT	STRENGTH	QUANTITY
Terbinafine tablets	250 mg	20
Ora-Plus:Simple syrup	1:1	qs 200 mL

NOTE: In this study, the formulation was stored in amber polyethylene prescription bottles.

INSTRUCTIONS: Crush the tablets in a mortar and triturate to a fine powder. Add small amounts of the vehicle and levigate to a uniform paste. Add vehicle almost to volume while mixing. Transfer to a graduate and qs to volume with vehicle.

NOTES

GENERIC NAME	**Terbutaline**
DOSAGE FORM	oral suspension
MADE FROM	tablets
CONCENTRATION	1 mg/mL
STABILITY	30 days
STABILITY REFERENCE	Abdel-Rahman SM, et al. Am J Hosp Pharm 1991;48:293-5
STORE	refrigerate
LABEL	shake well before use, refrigerate

INGREDIENT	STRENGTH	QUANTITY
Terbutaline sulfate tablets	5 mg	24
Purified water, USP		5 mL
Simple syrup, NF		qs 120 mL

NOTE: In this study, the formulation was stored in amber-colored type III glass prescription bottles.

INSTRUCTIONS: Crush the tablets in a glass mortar and triturate to a fine powder. Levigate with water into a smooth paste. Add approximately 30 mL of simple syrup in geometric proportions, mix thoroughly, and transfer to a graduate. Rinse the mortar with approximately 30 mL of the syrup, transfer to the graduate, and qs to 120 mL.

NOTES

GENERIC NAME	**Tetracycline**
DOSAGE FORM	oral suspension
MADE FROM	capsules
CONCENTRATION	25 mg/mL
STABILITY	7 days
STABILITY REFERENCE	Allen LV, et al. Am J Health Syst Pharm 1998; 55:1804-9
STORE	refrigerate
LABEL	shake well before use, refrigerate

INGREDIENT	STRENGTH	QUANTITY
Tetracycline hydrochloride capsules	500 mg	6
Cherry syrup (cherry syrup concentrate diluted 1:4 with simple syrup, NF)		qs 120 mL

NOTE:	In this study, the formulation was stored in amber clear plastic (polyethylene terephthalate) prescription ovals. Commercially available as an oral solution, 125 mg/5 mL.
INSTRUCTIONS:	Empty the contents of the capsules into a mortar and triturate to a fine powder. Add approximately 20 mL of the vehicle and levigate to a uniform paste. Add vehicle in geometric proportions almost to volume, mix thoroughly, and transfer to a graduate. Rinse the mortar with vehicle, add to the graduate, and qs to 120 mL.

NOTES

Copyright © 2011 Harvey Whitney Books

GENERIC NAME	**Tetracycline**
DOSAGE FORM	oral suspension
MADE FROM	capsules
CONCENTRATION	25 mg/mL
STABILITY	10 days
STABILITY REFERENCE	Allen LV, et al. Am J Health Syst Pharm 1998;55:1804-9
STORE	refrigerate
LABEL	shake well before use, refrigerate

INGREDIENT	STRENGTH	QUANTITY
Tetracycline hydrochloride capsules	500 mg	6
Ora-Plus:Ora-Sweet SF	(1:1)	qs 120 mL

NOTE: In this study, the formulation was stored in amber clear plastic (polyethylene terephthalate) prescription ovals. Commercially available as an oral solution, 125 mg/5 mL.

INSTRUCTIONS: Empty the contents of the capsules into a mortar and triturate to a fine powder. Add approximately 20 mL of the vehicle and levigate to a uniform paste. Add vehicle in geometric proportions almost to volume, mix thoroughly, and transfer to a graduate. Rinse the mortar with vehicle, add to the graduate, and qs to 120 mL.

NOTES

GENERIC NAME	**Tetracycline**
DOSAGE FORM	oral suspension
MADE FROM	capsules
CONCENTRATION	25 mg/mL
STABILITY	28 days
STABILITY REFERENCE	Allen LV, et al. Am J Health Syst Pharm 1998; 55:1804-9
STORE	refrigerate (preferable) or at room temperature
LABEL	shake well before use, refrigerate

INGREDIENT	STRENGTH	QUANTITY
Tetracycline hydrochloride capsules	500 mg	6
Ora-Plus and Ora-Sweet	(1:1)	qs 120 mL

NOTE: In this study, the formulation was stored in amber clear plastic (polyethylene terephthalate) prescription ovals. Commercially available as an oral solution, 125 mg/5 mL.

INSTRUCTIONS: Empty the contents of the capsules into a mortar and triturate to a fine powder. Add approximately 20 mL of the vehicle and levigate to a uniform paste. Add vehicle in geometric proportions almost to volume, mix thoroughly, and transfer to a graduate. Rinse the mortar with vehicle, add to the graduate, and qs to 120 mL.

NOTES

Copyright © 2011 Harvey Whitney Books

GENERIC NAME	**Tetracycline**
DOSAGE FORM	ophthalmic ointment
MADE FROM	powder
CONCENTRATION	1%
STABILITY	6 months
STABILITY REFERENCE	Tetracycline hydrochloride 1% ophthalmic ointment. Int J Pharmaceut Compd 2001;5:212
STORE	room temperature
LABEL	for ophthalmic use only

INGREDIENT	STRENGTH	QUANTITY
Tetracycline hydrochloride	1 g	
Mineral oil		1 g
White petrolatum		98 g

NOTE: Sterility testing not performed. Stability-indicating analytical methods not used. Based on *United States Pharmacopeia XXIV/National Formulary 19* (Rockville, MD: US Pharmacopeial Convention, 1999:2698-702) beyond-use date recommendation.

INSTRUCTIONS: Sterilize the white petrolatum and mineral oil by means of dry heat. Dissolve tetracycline in a sufficient amount of absolute alcohol (~110 mL) to form a clear solution. Filter the solution through a 0.2-µm filter needle into a sterile beaker under a laminar flow hood. Allow the beaker containing the alcohol to remain in the hood until the alcohol has evaporated. Using aseptic technique and sterile apparatus, levigate the sterile powder into the sterile mineral oil to form a smooth paste. Levigate the white petrolatum into the smooth paste in geometric proportions to form a uniform mixture. Transfer into sterile, light-resistant ophthalmic ointment tubes or into sterile syringes without needles. American Society of Health-System Pharmacists' guidelines (Am J Hosp Pharm 1993;50:1462-3) for compounding ophthalmic products should be considered while preparing this formulation.

NOTES

GENERIC NAME	**Thioguanine**
DOSAGE FORM	oral suspension
MADE FROM	tablets
CONCENTRATION	40 mg/mL
STABILITY	84 days
STABILITY REFERENCE	Dressman JB, et al. Am J Hosp Pharm 1983;40: 616-8
STORE	refrigerate (preferable) or at room temperature
LABEL	shake well before use, refrigerate

INGREDIENT	STRENGTH	QUANTITY
Thioguanine tablets	40 mg	15
Methylcellulose solution	1%	10 mL
Simple syrup, NF		qs 30 mL

NOTE: Stability-indicating analytical methods not used. In this study, the formulation contained Cologel 33 mL and wild cherry syrup:simple syrup, NF (1:2) qs 100 mL of 20 mg/mL of the formulation. Cologel, a commercially available vehicle consisting of methylcellulose 9% solution, is no longer available. In the above formulation, Cologel can be substituted with methylcellulose 1% solution and the wild cherry syrup:simple syrup mixture with simple syrup, NF.

INSTRUCTIONS: Crush the tablets and triturate to a fine powder. Make a mixture of equal parts of syrup and methylcellulose. Add a small amount of this vehicle and levigate to a uniform paste. Add the vehicle in geometric proportions almost to volume, mix thoroughly, and transfer to a graduate. Rinse the mortar with vehicle, add to the graduate, and qs to 30 mL.

NOTES

GENERIC NAME	**Three Bromides Syrup**
DOSAGE FORM	oral syrup
MADE FROM	crystals
CONCENTRATION	0.96 g/4 mL
STABILITY	12 months
STABILITY REFERENCE	experience
STORE	refrigerate
LABEL	refrigerate

INGREDIENT	STRENGTH	QUANTITY
Ammonium bromide crystals		8 g
Potassium bromide crystals		8 g
Sodium bromide crystals		8 g
Ora-Sweet		qs ad 100 mL

INSTRUCTIONS: Weigh the bromide crystals and add to 80 mL of the Ora-Sweet syrup in a graduate. Stir until dissolved (slowly soluble) and qs to 100 mL with Ora-Sweet syrup.

NOTES

GENERIC NAME	**Tiagabine**
DOSAGE FORM	oral suspension
MADE FROM	tablets
CONCENTRATION	1 mg/mL
STABILITY	91 days (4 °C); 42 days (25 °C)
STABILITY REFERENCE	Nahata MC, et al. Presented at: American Society of Health-System Pharmacists Midyear Clinical Meeting, Las Vegas, December 3–7, 2000 (poster)
STORE	refrigerate (preferable) or at room temperature
LABEL	shake well before use, refrigerate

INGREDIENT	STRENGTH	QUANTITY
Tiagabine tablets	12 mg	10
Methylcellulose	1%	17 mL
Simple syrup, NF		qs 120 mL

NOTE: In this study, the formulation was stored in plastic prescription bottles.

INSTRUCTIONS: Crush the tablets and triturate to mix well. Levigate the powder with methylcellulose gel to obtain a uniform paste. Add syrup in geometric proportions, mix well, and transfer to a graduate. Rinse the mortar with syrup, transfer to graduate, and qs to 120 mL.

NOTES

GENERIC NAME	**Tiagabine**
DOSAGE FORM	oral suspension
MADE FROM	tablets
CONCENTRATION	1 mg/mL
STABILITY	91 days (4 °C); 70 days (25 °C)
STABILITY REFERENCE	Nahata MC, et al. Presented at: American Society of Health-System Pharmacists Midyear Clinical Meeting, Las Vegas, December 3–7, 2000 (poster)
STORE	refrigerate (preferable) or at room temperature
LABEL	shake well before use, refrigerate

INGREDIENT	STRENGTH	QUANTITY
Tiagabine tablets	12 mg	10
Ora-Plus:Ora-Sweet	1:1	qs 120 mL

NOTE: In this study, the formulation was stored in plastic prescription bottles.

INSTRUCTIONS: Crush the tablets and triturate to mix well. Levigate the powder with the vehicle to obtain a uniform paste. Add vehicle in geometric proportions, mix well, and transfer to a graduate. Rinse the mortar with vehicle, transfer to graduate, and qs to 120 mL.

NOTES

GENERIC NAME	**Tobramycin**
DOSAGE FORM	ophthalmic drops
MADE FROM	injection
CONCENTRATION	15 mg/mL
STABILITY	28 days
STABILITY REFERENCE	Bowe BE, et al. Am J Ophthalmol 1991;111:686-9
STORE	refrigerate (preferable) or at room temperature
LABEL	refrigerate, for ophthalmic use only

INGREDIENT	STRENGTH	QUANTITY
Tobramycin sulfate injection (lyophilized, preservative-free)	40 mg/mL	
Methylcellulose artificial tears		qs to reconstitute

NOTE: Sterility testing not performed. Stability-indicating analytical methods not used.

INSTRUCTIONS: Reconstitute the injection with the artificial tears under a laminar air flow hood, using aseptic technique to achieve a concentration of 15 mg/mL. Transfer the solution to sterile ophthalmic dropper bottles. American Society of Health-System Pharmacists' guidelines (Am J Hosp Pharm 1993;50:1462-3) for compounding ophthalmic products should be considered while preparing this formulation.

NOTES

GENERIC NAME	**Tobramycin**
DOSAGE FORM	ophthalmic drops
MADE FROM	injection
CONCENTRATION	15 mg/mL
STABILITY	28 days
STABILITY REFERENCE	Charlton JF, et al. Am J Health Syst Pharm 1998;55:463-6
STORE	refrigerate (preferable) or at room temperature
LABEL	refrigerate, for ophthalmic use only

INGREDIENT	STRENGTH	QUANTITY
Tobramycin sulfate injection	40 mg/mL	3.75 mL
Artificial tears (Liquifilm Tears)		6.25 mL

NOTE: Sterility testing not performed. Stability-indicating analytical methods not used.

INSTRUCTIONS: Under the laminar air flow hood, withdraw the artificial tears from the bottle, using aseptic technique, to retain 6.25 mL. Add 3.75 mL of tobramycin sulfate solution to the original artificial tears bottle. Mix well. American Society of Health-System Pharmacists' guidelines (Am J Hosp Pharm 1993;50:1462-3) for compounding ophthalmic products should be considered while preparing this formulation.

NOTES

GENERIC NAME	**Tobramycin, Fortified**
DOSAGE FORM	ophthalmic drops
MADE FROM	injection
CONCENTRATION	13.6 mg/mL
STABILITY	90 days (4–8 °C)
STABILITY REFERENCE	McBride HA, et al. Am J Hosp Pharm 1991;48: 507-8
STORE	refrigerate
LABEL	refrigerate, for ophthalmic use only

INGREDIENT	STRENGTH	QUANTITY
Tobramycin ophthalmic solution (Tobrex)	3 mg/mL	5 mL
Tobramycin sulfate injection (lyophilized, preservative-free)	40 mg/mL	2 mL

NOTE: Sterility testing not performed.

INSTRUCTIONS: Add 2 mL of 40 mg/mL injectable solution to 5 mL of 3 mg/mL ophthalmic solution under a laminar air flow hood using aseptic techniques. American Society of Health-System Pharmacists' guidelines (Am J Hosp Pharm 1993;50:1462-3) for compounding ophthalmic products should be considered while preparing this formulation.

NOTES

GENERIC NAME	**Topiramate**
DOSAGE FORM	oral suspension
MADE FROM	tablets
CONCENTRATION	6 mg/mL
STABILITY	90 days
STABILITY REFERENCE	Nahata MC, et al. Presented at: American Society of Health-System Pharmacists Midyear Clinical Meeting, New Orleans, December 2–6, 2001 (poster)
STORE	refrigerate (preferable) or at room temperature
LABEL	shake well before use, refrigerate

INGREDIENT	STRENGTH	QUANTITY
Topiramate tablets	100 mg	6
Ora-Plus:Ora-Sweet	1:1	qs 100 mL

NOTE: In this study, the formulation was stored in plastic prescription bottles.

INSTRUCTIONS: Crush the tablets and triturate to a fine powder in a mortar. Levigate the powder with the vehicle into a uniform paste. Add vehicle in geometric proportions with constant mixing and transfer to a graduate. Rinse the mortar with the vehicle, transfer to the graduate, and qs to 100 mL.

NOTES

Copyright © 2011 Harvey Whitney Books

GENERIC NAME	**Topiramate**
DOSAGE FORM	oral suspension
MADE FROM	tablets
CONCENTRATION	6 mg/mL
STABILITY	90 days
STABILITY REFERENCE	Nahata MC, et al. Presented at: American Society of Health-System Pharmacists Midyear Clinical Meeting, New Orleans, December 2–6, 2001 (poster)
STORE	refrigerate (preferable) or at room temperature
LABEL	shake well before use, refrigerate

INGREDIENT	STRENGTH	QUANTITY
Topiramate tablets	100 mg	6
Methylcellulose 1% with parabens		10 mL
Simple syrup, NF		qs 100 mL

NOTE: In this study, the formulation was stored in plastic prescription bottles.

INSTRUCTIONS: Crush the tablets and triturate to a fine powder in a mortar. Levigate the powder with methylcellulose gel into a uniform paste. Add simple syrup in geometric proportions with constant mixing and transfer to a graduate. Rinse the mortar with syrup, transfer to the graduate, and qs to 100 mL.

NOTES

GENERIC NAME	**Trimethoprim**
DOSAGE FORM	oral suspension
MADE FROM	tablets
CONCENTRATION	10 mg/mL
STABILITY	91 days (4 °C); 42 days (25 °C)
STABILITY REFERENCE	Nahata MC, et al. J Pediatr Pharm Pract 1997;2:82-4
STORE	refrigerate
LABEL	shake well before use, refrigerate

INGREDIENT	STRENGTH	QUANTITY
Trimethoprim tablets	100 mg	10
Simple syrup, NF: methylcellulose 1% (50:50 v/v)	1:1	qs 100 mL

NOTE: In this study, the formulation was stored in plastic and glass prescription bottles. Commercially available as an oral solution, 50 mg/5 mL.

INSTRUCTIONS: Crush the tablets in a mortar and triturate to a fine powder. Add approximately 20 mL of vehicle and levigate to a uniform paste. Add 50 mL of the vehicle in geometric proportions, mix thoroughly, and transfer to a graduate. Rinse the mortar with the remaining vehicle, add to the graduate, and qs to 100 mL.

NOTES

GENERIC NAME	**Trimethoprim**
DOSAGE FORM	oral suspension
MADE FROM	tablets
CONCENTRATION	10 mg/mL
STABILITY	91 days
STABILITY REFERENCE	experience
STORE	refrigerate
LABEL	shake well before use, refrigerate

INGREDIENT	STRENGTH	QUANTITY
Trimethoprim tablet	100 mg	1
Simple syrup, NF:methyl-cellulose 1%	1:1	qs ad 10 mL

INSTRUCTIONS: Crush the tablet in a mortar. Add the vehicle gradually while mixing.

NOTES

GENERIC NAME	**Ursodiol**
DOSAGE FORM	oral suspension
MADE FROM	capsules
CONCENTRATION	60 mg/mL
STABILITY	35 days
STABILITY REFERENCE	Johnson CE, et al. Am J Health Syst Pharm 1995;52:1798-800
STORE	refrigerate
LABEL	shake well before use, refrigerate

INGREDIENT	STRENGTH	QUANTITY
Ursodiol capsules	300 mg	12
Glycerin, USP		qs to wet the powder
Simple syrup, NF		qs 60 mL

NOTE: In this study, the formulation was stored in type III amber glass prescription bottles.

INSTRUCTIONS: Empty the contents of the capsules into a mortar and triturate to mix thoroughly. Add a small amount of glycerin to wet the powder and levigate into a smooth paste. Add approximately 15 mL of syrup in geometric proportions, mix thoroughly, and transfer to a graduate. Rinse the mortar with approximately 15 mL of syrup and transfer to the graduate. Repeat the above steps and add enough syrup to qs to 60 mL.

NOTES

GENERIC NAME	**Ursodiol**
DOSAGE FORM	oral suspension
MADE FROM	capsules
CONCENTRATION	20 mg/mL
STABILITY	91 days
STABILITY REFERENCE	Nahata MC, et al. J Appl Ther Res 1999;2:221-4
STORE	refrigerate (preferable) or at room temperature
LABEL	shake well before use, refrigerate

INGREDIENT	STRENGTH	QUANTITY
Ursodiol capsules	300 mg	17
Ora-Sweet/Ora-Plus or methylcellulose 1%/ simple syrup, NF	1:1 mixture	qs 255 mL

NOTE: In this study, the formulation was stored in amber plastic prescription bottles.

INSTRUCTIONS: Empty the contents of the capsules into a mortar and reduce to a fine powder. Add a small amount of the vehicle to the powder and mix to a uniform paste. Add geometric proportions of the vehicle almost to volume. Transfer to a graduate and qs to 255 mL with vehicle while mixing.

NOTES

GENERIC NAME	**Ursodiol**
DOSAGE FORM	oral suspension
MADE FROM	capsules
CONCENTRATION	25 mg/mL
STABILITY	60 days (at 2–6 °C and at 22–23 °C)
STABILITY REFERENCE	Mallet MS, et al. Am J Health Syst Pharm 1997;54:1401-4
STORE	refrigerate (preferable) or at room temperature
LABEL	shake well before use, refrigerate

INGREDIENT	STRENGTH	QUANTITY
Ursodiol capsules	300 mg	10
Glycerin, USP		10 mL
Ora-Plus		60 mL
Orange syrup, NF		qs 120 mL

NOTE: In this study, the formulation was stored in amber plastic prescription bottles.

INSTRUCTIONS: Empty the contents of the capsules into a mortar and triturate to mix thoroughly. Add glycerin and levigate into a smooth paste. Add 60 mL of Ora-Plus in geometric proportions, mix thoroughly, and transfer to a graduate. Rinse the mortar with approximately 30 mL of orange syrup and transfer to the graduate. Repeat the above steps and add enough syrup to qs to 120 mL.

NOTES

GENERIC NAME	**Valacyclovir**
DOSAGE FORM	oral suspension
MADE FROM	caplets
CONCENTRATION	50 mg/mL
STABILITY	21 days
STABILITY REFERENCE	Fish DN, et al. Am J Health Syst Pharm 1999;56: 1957-60
STORE	refrigerate
LABEL	shake well before use, refrigerate

INGREDIENT	STRENGTH	QUANTITY
Valacyclovir caplets	500 mg	18
Ora-Sweet or Ora-Sweet SF or syspalta		qs 180 mL

NOTE: In this study, the formulation was stored in amber glass bottles.

INSTRUCTIONS: Crush the caplets in a mortar and reduce to a fine powder. Add 40 mL of Ora-Sweet in small increments to the powder, mixing thoroughly. Pour the resulting mixture into a graduate. Rinse the mortar with Ora-Sweet or Ora-Sweet SF while mixing, then qs the mixture to 180 mL.

NOTES

GENERIC NAME	**Verapamil**
DOSAGE FORM	oral suspension
MADE FROM	tablets
CONCENTRATION	50 mg/mL
STABILITY	60 days
STABILITY REFERENCE	Allen LV Jr, et al. Am J Health Syst Pharm 1996;53:2304-8
STORE	refrigerate (preferable) or at room temperature
LABEL	shake well before use, refrigerate

INGREDIENT	STRENGTH	QUANTITY
Verapamil hydrochloride tablets	80 mg	75
Cherry syrup (cherry syrup concentrate diluted 1:4 with simple syrup, NF)		qs 120 mL

NOTE: In this study, the formulation was stored in amber clear plastic (polyethylene terephthalate) prescription ovals.

INSTRUCTIONS: Crush the tablets and triturate to a fine powder. Add approximately 20 mL of the vehicle and levigate to a uniform paste. Add the vehicle in geometric proportions almost to volume, mix thoroughly, and transfer to a graduate. Rinse the mortar with vehicle, add to the graduate, and qs to 120 mL.

NOTES

GENERIC NAME	**Verapamil**
DOSAGE FORM	oral suspension
MADE FROM	tablets
CONCENTRATION	50 mg/mL
STABILITY	91 days
STABILITY REFERENCE	Nahata MC. J Appl Ther Res 1997;1:271-3
STORE	refrigerate (preferable) or at room temperature
LABEL	shake well before use, refrigerate

INGREDIENT	STRENGTH	QUANTITY
Verapamil tablets	80 mg	20
Purified water, USP		3 mL
Methylcellulose 1%:simple syrup, NF	1:1	qs 32 mL

NOTE: In this study, the formulation was stored in plastic and glass prescription bottles.

INSTRUCTIONS: Pulverize the tablets in a mortar. Add water and triturate until a smooth paste is formed. Add the vehicle and mix. Transfer to a graduate and qs to volume with the vehicle.

NOTES

GENERIC NAME	**Verapamil**
DOSAGE FORM	oral suspension
MADE FROM	tablets
CONCENTRATION	50 mg/mL
STABILITY	60 days
STABILITY REFERENCE	Allen LV Jr, et al. Am J Health Syst Pharm 1996; 53:2304-8
STORE	refrigerate (preferable) or at room temperature
LABEL	shake well before use, refrigerate

INGREDIENT	STRENGTH	QUANTITY
Verapamil tablets	80 mg	75
Ora-Plus:Ora-Sweet	1:1	
or Ora-Plus:Ora-Sweet SF		qs 120 mL

NOTE: In this study, the formulation was stored in amber plastic (polyethylene terephthalate) prescription ovals.

INSTRUCTIONS: Crush the tablets in a mortar and reduce to a fine powder. Add a small amount of vehicle and mix to a uniform paste. Add geometric amounts of vehicle almost to desired volume while mixing. Transfer to a graduate and qs to volume while mixing.

NOTES

GENERIC NAME	**Voriconazole**
DOSAGE FORM	oral suspension
MADE FROM	tablets
CONCENTRATION	40 mg/mL
STABILITY	30 days
STABILITY REFERENCE	Nguyen KQ, et al. Am J Vet Res 2009;70:908-14
STORE	refrigerate (preferable) or room temperature
LABEL	shake well before use, refrigerate

INGREDIENT	STRENGTH	QUANTITY
Voriconazole tablets	200 mg	8
Deionized water		10 mL
Ora-Plus		30 mL

NOTE: In this study, the formulation was stored in amber-colored plastic bottles.

INSTRUCTIONS: Mix deionized water and Ora-Plus in geometric proportions with constant stirring to produce 40 mL. Triturate eight tablets into a fine powder in a glass mortar. Using 10 mL of this mixture levigate the powder into a smooth suspension, adding the vehicle in geometric proportions. Transfer the suspension to a graduate. Rinse the mortar with sufficient vehicle to bring the final volume in the bottle to 40 mL.

NOTES

GENERIC NAME	**Voriconazole**
DOSAGE FORM	oral suspension
MADE FROM	tablets
CONCENTRATION	40 mg/mL
STABILITY	30 days
STABILITY REFERENCE	Nguyen KQ, et al. Am J Vet Res 2009;70:908-14
STORE	refrigerate or room temperature
LABEL	shake well before use, refrigerate

INGREDIENT	STRENGTH	QUANTITY
Voriconazole tablets	200 mg	8
Ora-Plus		20 mL
Ora-Sweet		20 mL

NOTE: In this study, the formulation was stored in amber-colored plastic bottles.

INSTRUCTIONS: Mix Ora-Plus and Ora-Sweet in geometric proportions with constant stirring to produce 40 mL. Triturate eight tablets into a fine powder in a glass mortar. Using 10 mL of this mixture levigate the powder into a smooth suspension, adding the vehicle in geometric proportions. Transfer the suspension to a graduate. Rinse the mortar with sufficient vehicle to bring the final volume in the bottle to 40 mL.

NOTES

GENERIC NAME	**Zinc Acetate**
DOSAGE FORM	oral syrup
MADE FROM	powder
CONCENTRATION	10 mg/mL elemental zinc
STABILITY	60 days
STABILITY REFERENCE	experience
STORE	refrigerate
LABEL	shake well before use, refrigerate

INGREDIENT	STRENGTH	QUANTITY
Zinc acetate powder		3.36 g
Purified water, USP		20 mL
Simple syrup, NF		qs ad 100 mL

INSTRUCTIONS: Dissolve the zinc acetate powder in 20 mL of water. Transfer to a graduate and qs to volume with syrup.

NOTES

GENERIC NAME	**Zonisamide**
DOSAGE FORM	oral suspension
MADE FROM	capsules
CONCENTRATION	10 mg/mL
STABILITY	91 days
STABILITY REFERENCE	Nahata MC, et al. Presented at: American Society of Health-System Pharmacists Midyear Clinical Meeting, December 2004 (poster)
STORE	refrigerate or room temperature
LABEL	refrigerate, shake well before use

INGREDIENT	STRENGTH	QUANTITY
Zonisamide capsules	100 mg	12
Simple syrup, NF: 1% methylcellulose suspension	1:10	qs 120 mL

NOTE: This formulation was stored in amber prescription bottles.
INSTRUCTIONS: Mix simple syrup and 1% methylcellulose suspension together thoroughly in a glass mortar, in geometric proportions, to prepare the vehicle. Triturate the tablets into a fine powder and levigate with small proportion of the vehicle into a smooth suspension. Add vehicle in geometric proportions, with constant mixing. Transfer to a graduate. Rinse the mortar with sufficient vehicle and transfer to graduate to make up the final volume.

NOTES

GENERIC NAME	**Zonisamide**
DOSAGE FORM	oral suspension
MADE FROM	capsules
CONCENTRATION	10 mg/mL
STABILITY	91 days
STABILITY REFERENCE	Nahata MC, et al. Presented at: American Society of Health-System Pharmacists Midyear Clinical Meeting, December 2004
STORE	refrigerate or room temperature
LABEL	refrigerate, protect from light, shake well before use

INGREDIENT	STRENGTH	QUANTITY
Zonisamide capsules	100 mg	6
Ora-Plus:Ora-Sweet	1:1	qs 120 mL

NOTE: This formulation was stored in amber prescription bottles.
INSTRUCTIONS: Mix Ora-Plus and Ora-Sweet together thoroughly in a glass mortar, in geometric proportions, to prepare the vehicle. Triturate the tablets into a fine powder and levigate with small proportion of the vehicle into a smooth suspension. Add vehicle in geometric proportions with constant mixing. Transfer to a graduate. Rinse the mortar with sufficient vehicle and transfer to graduate to make up the final volume.

NOTES

GENERIC NAME	**Zonisamide**
DOSAGE FORM	oral suspension
MADE FROM	capsules
CONCENTRATION	10 mg/mL
STABILITY	7 days
STABILITY REFERENCE	Abobo CV, et al. Am J Health Syst Pharm 2009;66:1105-9
STORE	room temperature
LABEL	protect from light, shake well before use

INGREDIENT	STRENGTH	QUANTITY
Zonisamide capsules	100 mg	12
Simple syrup, NF		qs 120 mL

NOTE: This formulation was stored in amber plastic prescription bottles.

INSTRUCTIONS: Open the capsules into a glass mortar and triturate the contents into a fine powder; levigate with small proportion of the syrup into a smooth suspension. Add syrup, in geometric proportions, with constant mixing. Transfer to a graduate. Rinse the mortar with sufficient vehicle and transfer to graduate to make up the final volume.

NOTES

GENERIC NAME	**Zonisamide**
DOSAGE FORM	oral suspension
MADE FROM	capsules
CONCENTRATION	10 mg/mL
STABILITY	14 days
STABILITY REFERENCE	Abobo CV, et al. Am J Health Syst Pharm 2009;66:1105-9
STORE	room temperature
LABEL	protect from light, shake well before use

INGREDIENT	STRENGTH	QUANTITY
Zonisamide capsules	100 mg	12
Methylcellulose suspension	0.5%	qs 120 mL

NOTE: This formulation was stored in amber plastic prescription bottles.

INSTRUCTIONS: Open the capsules into a glass mortar and triturate the contents into a fine powder; levigate with small proportion of the vehicle into a smooth suspension. Add the vehicle, in geometric proportions, with constant mixing. Transfer to a graduate. Rinse the mortar with sufficient vehicle and transfer to graduate to make up the final volume.

NOTES

GENERIC NAME

DOSAGE FORM

MADE FROM

CONCENTRATION

STABILITY

STABILITY REFERENCE

STORE

LABEL

INGREDIENT	STRENGTH	QUANTITY

INSTRUCTIONS:

GENERIC NAME

DOSAGE FORM

MADE FROM

CONCENTRATION

STABILITY

STABILITY REFERENCE

STORE

LABEL

INGREDIENT	STRENGTH	QUANTITY

INSTRUCTIONS:

GENERIC NAME

DOSAGE FORM

MADE FROM

CONCENTRATION

STABILITY

STABILITY REFERENCE

STORE

LABEL

INGREDIENT	STRENGTH	QUANTITY

INSTRUCTIONS:

GENERIC NAME

DOSAGE FORM

MADE FROM

CONCENTRATION

STABILITY

STABILITY REFERENCE

STORE

LABEL

INGREDIENT	STRENGTH	QUANTITY

NOTE: Text
INSTRUCTIONS: Text

NOTES

Copyright © 2011 Harvey Whitney Books

FEEDBACK FORM

Use this form to send us your formulations or comments regarding the formulations published in this book. Please photocopy this form and submit one form per formulation. Please include your name, the name and address of your institution, your telephone and fax numbers, and your E-mail address with your correspondence.

Mail this form to Harvey Whitney Books Company, P.O. Box 42696, Cincinnati, OH 45242 USA or fax to 513/793-3600. Or, you may complete this form online at www.hwbooks.com and include any other comments, corrections, or suggestions.

GENERIC NAME

DOSAGE FORM

MADE FROM

CONCENTRATION

STABILITY

STABILITY REFERENCE

STORE

LABEL

INGREDIENT	STRENGTH	QUANTITY

INSTRUCTIONS:

Copyright © 2011 Harvey Whitney Books